Michele Sharp is the
director of development and communica-
tions for The Migraine Association of Canada
and has volunteered or worked in the not for-
profit sector for most of her life. She works
with migraine sufferers daily, helping to fos-
ter a greater understanding of the disorder
through education, support, and empowerment. She lives in Canada.

THE Migraine COOKBOOK

{ More Than 100 Healthy and Delicious
Recipes for Migraine Sufferers }

Michele Sharp

MARLOWE & COMPANY

THE MIGRAINE COOKBOOK:
More Than 100 Healthy and Delicious Recipes for Migraine Sufferers
Copyright © 2001, 2002 by Michele Sharp

Published by
Marlowe & Company
An Imprint of Avalon Publishing Group Incorporated
161 William Street, 16th Floor
New York, NY 10038

Originally published in Canada by Key Porter Books Limited.
This edition published by arrangement.

Library of Congress Control Number:
2002100743

9   8   7   6   5   4   3   2   1

DESIGNED BY PAULINE NEUWIRTH, NEUWIRTH & ASSOCIATES, INC.

Printed in the United States of America
Distributed by Publishers Group West

Contents

Meatless Main Courses

Meat and Poultry

Fish and Seafood

Vegetables and Side Dishes

Basic Stocks and Sauces

Quick Breads

Desserts and Baked Goods

Beverages

Foreword

Migraine is one of the most undertreated, misunderstood, and misdiagnosed disorders of the past century. And yet it is a serious medical disorder that significantly affects millions of North Americans. In fact, prevalence studies indicate that 15 to 18 percent of women, 5 to 6 percent of men, 4 to 5 percent of children under twelve, and 10 percent of adolescents suffer from this disorder. As Rosemary Dudley, the founder of The Migraine Association of Canada, stated, "Perhaps no other condition so disrupts the lives of its victims and yet evokes so little sympathy and compassion for the afflicted."

As Rosemary's comment suggests, migraine has a significant impact on an individual's personal and professional life. It can lead to lost workdays, hindered job performance, restricted activities, and disrupted relationships. A U.S. study estimates that 112 million bedridden days a year cost U.S. employers as much as $13 billion, and the U.S. economy $1 billion in direct medical costs.

While there is no known cure for migraine, understanding your triggers can help you take charge of your attacks. For those of you who find that certain foods can be a trigger, *The Migraine Cookbook* will help to educate and empower you. It has been designed to make you think more about your lifestyle so that you can recognize patterns that lead to an attack. Through identifying and eliminating or avoiding your triggers, I hope you will be able to provide yourself a measure of relief against the terrible pain of migraine.

The inspiration for this book must go first to our Fredericton, New Brunswick, chapter. They were a wonderful source for many of the delicious recipes. I would also like to individually thank those loyal members, volunteers, and supporters across Canada who provided support in bringing the various elements of this book together: Joanne Brown; Heather-Ann Brown; Erik

Buchanan; Bonnie Buxton; Elaine Comish; Maria Conforto; Pamela Douglas; Laura Eagle-LaDuke; Sylvia Fowles; Edith Freeman; Alice Gauvin; Patti Hanson; Laura Hennick; John Holland; Maura Keenan; Sally Ann Kerman; Lois Lavers; Sara Lawson; Emily Levitt; Meg Lloyd-Jones; Connie Luyt; Arlene Mahood; Elizabeth McKim; Ruth Miln; Victoria Mountain; Bob Olsen; Olga Peacock; Dr. Allan Purdy; Jenny Reid; Dr. Gordon Robinson; Mary-Ann Roebellen; Andrea Rolston; Bill Ross; Nelly Sabbagh; Malcolm Sharp; Nelda Sharp; Dr. Ashfaq Shuaib; Donna-Lynn Turner; G. Joy Underwood; Grace Wood; and Dave Wright. I'd also like to recognize our dedicated volunteer Board of Directors: Georgina Kossivas, Dr. Marek Gawel, Karen Ormerod, Barbara Nawrocki, Dr. Rose Giammario, Dr. Gary Shapero, and Debbie Drewett.

Special thanks should also go to Susan Folkins, my editor, for all her patience and advice. Thanks also to Anna Porter, Clare McKeon, Irene Worthington, Valerie South, Liba Berry, and Cathy Fraccaro. All of your comments, suggestions, and keen support were greatly appreciated.

I'd also like to recognize Astra Zeneca for their commitment to The Migraine Association of Canada and their assistance in making aspects of this project possible.

Many Toronto chefs generously contributed recipes to our first cookbook, *Fabulous Cooking Ideas*. Some of their recipes are reprinted here. Thanks also to the chefs at North 44 for sharing their delicious recipe for Steamed Basmati Rice with Crisp Potatoes, Sumac, and Cumin. I would also like to thank the authors of *HeartHealthy Cooking, Fare for Friends,* and *Good Friends Cookbook* for granting us permission to reprint a few of their recipes.

Finally, I would like to thank our invaluable volunteers who provided us with their time, energy, and support. We would not be able to continue to provide much-needed information, education, and services without you!

—MICHELE SHARP

More Than Just a Headache

Almost everyone gets a headache now and then. The most common form of headache is tension headache. Unlike migraine, tension headache is mild to moderate and is usually alleviated with rest and relaxation or over-the-counter pain relievers. Migraine, however, is a neurological disorder that involves a complex relationship between the blood supply to the brain and its nerve network.

Migraine occurs most often among people ages 20 to 50. The most common symptom is severe head pain made worse by routine activities such as climbing stairs or bending over. The pain, often described by sufferers as throbbing, is commonly felt on one side of the head, although it can switch sides during an attack or from one attack to the next. Many migraine sufferers feel nauseous, and some vomit during an attack. Typically, sufferers are extremely sensitive to light, sound, and odors, making ordinary events unbearable.

For the majority of migraine sufferers, an untreated or unsuccessfully treated attack lasts 24 hours, although attacks can vary from two hours to several days. An average sufferer may have as many as 20 attacks every year; however, as many as 9 percent of sufferers experience 52 or more. During an attack and often leading up to and following an attack, sufferers can become disabled; that is, they must completely or partially restrict their activities.

Migraine is more than a just a headache. In addition to waves of nausea and sensitivity to light, sound, and odors, about one-fifth of migraine sufferers experience an "aura," a visual or sensory disturbance that acts as a warning sign to the oncoming headache. Other symptoms often experienced in the period of time leading up to the headache include: irritability, depression, elation, excessive yawning, difficulty concentrating, dizziness, trouble with words, hyperactivity, and food cravings. (For more about the symptoms of migraine, see p. 11.)

{ Why People Get Migraines }

Experts have yet to pinpoint the exact cause of migraine, but they do know it tends to run in families. In fact, more than 50 percent of migraine sufferers have a close relative who experiences similar headaches, which indicates that migraine may be inherited. With the discovery of the gene responsible for familial hemiplegic migraine (a very rare form of the disorder), experts believe that further research may enable them to generalize this information to the broader disorder. In the meantime, leading health experts describe individuals with migraine as wired differently, with a predisposition toward episodic migraine attacks. What triggers individual attacks varies between people and from one attack to the next.

{ What Happens in the Head }

We do not have complete understanding of the complex chain of physical events that precipitate a migraine attack. However, research in the past few decades has led to a better understanding of what happens in the head during a migraine attack. Researchers now know that certain chemicals in the brain—substance P, neurokinin A, and calcitonin gene-related peptide (CGRP), among others—are released and land on blood vessels. These chemicals cause the blood vessels to expand and send signals via the nerves to the brain, where the signals are processed to determine that the sensation is a painful one.

{ Types of Migraine }

The two most common types of migraine are migraine without aura and migraine with aura. There are also several subtypes (atypical migraines) that are quite rare. They present themselves differently from the more common types, but researchers believe the triggers are the same.

MIGRAINE WITHOUT AURA (PREVIOUSLY CALLED "COMMON MIGRAINE")

Most people experience migraine without aura. The pain is usually described as throbbing and is made worse by routine activities such as climbing stairs or bending over. Pain is on one side of the head (although it can be on both sides or switch sides during an attack or from one attack to the next). Nausea and/or vomiting and extreme sensitivity to light, sound, or smell are other symptoms. People afflicted with migraine frequently describe the pain as "hammering" or "pulsating."

Migraine with aura (previously called "classic migraine")

As many as 20 percent of migraine sufferers experience an aura before their attack. An aura is a visual or sensory disturbance that acts as a warning sign of the oncoming headache. Typical aura symptoms include flashes of light, blurred vision, or blind spots spreading across the visual field. Some sufferers may feel tingling or numbness in the face, arms, or hands. These symptoms usually fade within an hour as they give way to severe head pain. In some cases, however, a headache never follows; some migraine sufferers have aura without headache.

Atypical migraine

There are also uncommon types of migraine such as familial hemiplegic migraine, basilar migraine, and ophthalmoplegic migraine.

Familial hemiplegic migraine is the only type of migraine to have had a specific gene identified. This very rare atypical migraine is believed to result from a prolonged and profound aura involving the brain. Symptoms often can mimic a stroke or tumor and range from a slight tingling or numbness on one side of the face or body to partial short-term paralysis. The headache is usually one-sided but the aftereffects of the aura can last for days. Rarely is it permanent.

Basilar migraine, also known as basilar artery migraine, Bickerstaff's migraine, and syncopal migraine, is associated with several distinct aura symptoms. They include:

- Visual symptoms such as double vision
- Slurred speech
- Dizziness and/or vertigo
- Ringing in the ears
- Decreased hearing
- Numbness and tingling in limbs on both sides or severe weakness/paralysis of limbs on both sides
- Decreased level of awareness of surroundings

Ophthalmoplegic migraine is a very rare type of migraine. It involves repeated headaches and a paralysis of one or more cranial nerves that control pupil dilation and eye movement. Sufferers often experience double vision, and the symptoms may be mistaken for an aneurysm (a ballooning of the blood vessels in the head that can rupture and cause bleeding).

OTHER TYPES OF HEADACHE

Medication-induced headaches/rebound headaches

Medication-induced headaches, or rebound headaches, have become increasingly common. Migraine sufferers are often susceptible to developing this condition. Scientists believe that when the level of analgesics (pain relievers) begins to lower in the body, the individual experiences a withdrawal reaction in the form of a headache. Increasing the level of analgesics relieves the headache, not because of the painkilling effect, but because it temporarily interrupts withdrawal. This condition can also occur with ergotamines. Only the complete elimination of analgesics or ergotamines from the system will end this vicious circle. Discuss the options with your doctor.

Cluster headaches

Cluster headaches, should not be confused with migraine attacks. Unlike migraine, which occurs in nearly 17 percent of the North American population, cluster headache occurs in less than 1 percent of the population. Eighty-five percent of all cluster headache sufferers are men.

The symptoms of cluster headache are distinctly different from those of migraine. Attacks of cluster headache are grouped in a series of short, intensely severe bursts of pain, usually lasting 30 to 45 minutes and rarely lasting longer than four hours. Often occurring at night, the pain is sharp, piercing, and debilitating. If you think you might be suffering from cluster headaches, consult your doctor and get a proper diagnosis. Cluster and migraine are two distinct disorders with different symptoms and treatments.

{ Migraine in Women }

Before puberty, the prevalence of migraine in both sexes is about equal. However, at the onset of puberty, the incidence of migraines in females increases dramatically. In adults, migraine is three times more prevalent in women than in men. It is believed that this is due to hormonal changes associated with the reproductive cycle.

For women whose migraines start at puberty, their migraines often show a lifelong connection to their menstrual cycle. Migraine attacks are linked to the menstrual cycle in about 60 percent of affected women (menstrually related migraine), and they are exclusive to the menstrual cycle in roughly 14 percent of affected women (true menstrual migraine). Both forms of menstrual migraine occur during or just after estrogen levels fall. Since estrogen levels fall after ovulation and before menstruation, this could account for headaches at these times. Depending on the woman's circumstances, doctors may prescribe hormone replacement therapy (HRT), which helps to stabilize estrogen levels during these critical times. In addition, some doctors prescribe nonsteroidal anti-inflammatory drugs (NSAIDs) such as ibuprofen or naproxen for the prevention of menstrual migraine.

For many women, their episodes of attacks lessen with pregnancy or menopause. But for some women, migraine may appear for the first time during pregnancy. Often it will improve during the second and third trimesters, but medication must be approached cautiously throughout pregnancy (especially the first trimester) and should be taken only on the advice of a doctor.

Oral contraceptives, which contain estrogen and progesterone, can induce, change, or alleviate migraine. Their use can trigger the first migraine attack (most often in women with a family history of migraine) or exacerbate existing migraine, especially on those days when the woman is off the oral contraceptive.

During the early menopausal stage, tremendous fluctuations in estrogen can worsen migraine. Hormone replacement with estrogen, alone or in combination with progesterone, can either exacerbate migraine or relieve it. Cyclical HRT may trigger migraine in the days off the supplement, so continuous low doses of estrogen and progesterone are sometimes preferable. In a recent North American study, about 62 percent of women experienced fewer migraine headaches and a marked improvement after menopause; 28 percent felt no difference; and 10 percent felt that their migraines were worse.

{ Migraine in Children }

If you're caring for a child with migraine, there may be some comfort in knowing that you're not alone. Approximately 4 to 5 percent of children suffer from migraine. While as many as one-third of children will outgrow migraine, many will go on to have it in adolescence. After age 12, the incidence of migraine increases in girls due to the role of hormones (see p. 13). By age 14, the rate for girls is approximately 15 percent, while the rate for boys hovers at 6 percent. Approximately 25 percent of adults with migraine report that their symptoms started before age 10.

Migraine in children is unique for several reasons. While identifying migraine in adults can be a challenge, diagnosing it in children is even more difficult. Children communicate their symptoms differently than adults. It's unlikely, for example, that you'll hear a child say, "I've been having a throbbing pain in my left temple accompanied by nausea two times a month." Instead, parents might notice that an otherwise playful child suddenly becomes introverted, irritable, or covers his or her eyes.

Naturally, migraine affects children in different ways than adults. Children may miss school, stop participating in social activities, decline invitations to parties, and, in some cases, may develop coping and communication problems. Adults caring for children with migraine can play a vital role in early detection, appropriate care, preventive measures, and the development of a support network—all of which contribute to a positive attitude toward the disorder and help enhance the sufferer's overall participation in life.

Sorting out the symptoms in children can be very difficult. As with adults, the most common form of migraine in children is migraine without aura, characterized by one or two-sided often frontal (across the forehead) moderate to severe head pain; sensitivity to light, sound and smells; and nausea or vomiting. Headaches in children are usually of shorter duration than those in adults. Your child's migraine may last for only one hour and may be relieved by a long nap. In some cases, it can last for as long as two days.

The second most common form, migraine with aura, is characterized by visual or sensory disturbances. Blind spots, difficulty focusing, and displays of flashing lights can be especially distressing for children. Other symptoms include numbness or tingling in the arms and hands or around the mouth. Some children will have the aura without headache, with the possibility of developing the headache later in life.

Additional symptoms, possibly indicative of other types of migraine, should be discussed with your doctor. These include double vision, eye pain, slurred speech, confusion, and weakness or paralysis. Very young children may experience abdominal pain, intense vomiting, loss of balance, or the feeling that everything around them is going very fast or very slow, or is unusually big or small. These symptoms may be the first expression of migraine and can frighten or confuse both the child and adult.

Getting an accurate diagnosis and ruling out other causes is the first step in managing migraine (see p. 10). Many symptoms will disappear as the child matures and grows out of them, or as the more common features of migraine become more prominent. A visit to the doctor to review the child's history and symptoms will establish whether the child has migraine.

The next step is identifying triggers. No two children have exactly the same triggers, although there are a number of common ones. Susceptibility to triggers will change from time to time, depending on the child's overall emotional and physical well-being. For some children, diet is a key trigger; for others, stress, missed sleep, skipped meals, changes in weather, or changes to routine can bring on migraine. Reducing exposure to triggers is a key strategy for reducing the frequency of migraine.

During migraine attacks, children may find comfort in retreating to a darkened, quiet room. Cold packs, fluids in moderation, and a short nap may stave off an attack. When nondrug strategies are not successful, medication is an option when used as directed. In pediatric doses, over-the-counter medications such as ibuprofen (for older children or adolescents) or acetaminophen can help alleviate an attack. Acetylsalicylic acid (ASA) should not be used in children 12 years and under because of its association with Reye's syndrome (an often fatal disease of the brain that usually occurs in children following an acute viral infection).

Combination pain relievers containing codeine or migraine-specific medications (such as sumatriptan, zolmitriptan, naratriptan, rizatriptan, or eletriptan) may be used in older children and adolescents when all other measures fail. Pain relievers should not be taken more than two days a week, in order to prevent rebound headaches (see p. 12). For chronic attacks or severe pain, emergency room treatment and/or preventive medications may be recommended.

In all cases, medication should be taken only at the advice of the child's physician. Some medications on the market have been tested only on adults and may not be suitable for children. Don't share your own or anyone else's medication with your child.

It is important to develop, as much as possible, nondrug strategies to cope with migraine, such as rest, relaxation, regular routines, and exercise. If tension or pressure at school or home is acting as a trigger, stress management, relaxation, biofeedback (see p. 15), hypnotherapy (see p. 23), or professional counseling can be effective. Developing early coping mechanisms will help your child deal effectively with migraine in the long run. As they say, an ounce of prevention is worth a pound of cure!

Diagnosis and Management of Migraine

Proper diagnosis of migraine is an important first step in taking control of your disorder. Many people (as many as 19 percent of sufferers) have never sought medical advice for their disorder, and as many as 45 percent lapse from physician care.

The next step to managing this disorder is to learn as much as possible about it and your triggers (whether they are dietary, hormonal, or stress- or environment-related) and to take steps to change your lifestyle.

{ Diagnosing Migraine }

First and foremost, managing migraine is about obtaining a diagnosis from a physician. According to a recent North American study, only 50 percent of migraine sufferers have actually been diagnosed and only 34 percent regularly consult a physician.

In 1988, the International Headache Society developed guidelines that considerably improved the diagnosis of migraine. Their diagnostic criteria for migraine included attacks lasting 4 to 72 hours, as well as some combination of the following symptoms:

- One-sided moderate to severe throbbing pain aggravated by movement
- Nausea or vomiting
- Sensitivity to light and sound
- Visual or sensory disturbances referred to as aura

WARNING SIGNS AND SYMPTOMS

Many people actually experience symptoms and do not realize that they could be part of migraine. These should be checked by a physician. In addition to the more easily recognized symptoms mentioned above, many people experience more subtle signs and symptoms with their attacks. These may be experienced prior to, as well as during, an attack and can include:

+ Dizziness
+ General discomfort in the stomach and/or abdominal area
+ Depression, irritability, tension, and/or other alteration in mood and outlook, sometimes with a feeling of detachment
+ Inability to concentrate
+ Feelings of extreme well-being with uncommon energy, vigor, and a feeling of excitement preceding the attack
+ Excessive yawning
+ Unusual hunger, and a desire for snacks, especially sweets
+ Talkativeness or difficulty forming words or recalling words and incidents
+ Pain or numbness in the neck and shoulder areas
+ Trembling
+ Patches or blotchy areas on the skin that look like a rash
+ Unusual paleness or pallor (especially true with children)
+ Increase in weight, perhaps along with swelling in the fingers and hands, waist, breasts, ankles, or legs, or an increase in frequency and volume of urination

These warning signs and symptoms are most frequently noted by physicians and those who suffer from migraine. They are sometimes called symptoms of the "prodrome" or aura. Some individuals have suggested other symptoms that are peculiar to them. As with the more easily recognized symptoms of migraine, not everyone experiences all of these symptoms. When you talk to your physician, it will help if you list your specific symptoms.

{ Triggers }

A trigger is any internal or external influence that activates or aggravates a migraine attack. Most people find that a combination of triggers brings on an attack. Because people afflicted with migraine are sensitive to these influences, it is important to identify triggers and reduce or eliminate their impact as much as possible. It is also important to remember that triggers in and of themselves are not the cause of migraine and that migraine is a complicated biological disorder.

If you can readily identify your triggers, you will find it much easier to manage your migraine attacks. You can eliminate or avoid some triggers, reduce others, and brace for those over which you have no control. While some triggers, such as weather, are not controllable, they often work in combination with those that are controllable, such as food. For this reason, simply being aware of them will help you to manage your migraine.

Keeping a diary will help you isolate your triggers. If you document your migraine attacks over a period of several months, you will probably notice that there is a pattern to your attacks. You should track the following items:

- Frequency of attacks
- Duration of attacks
- What the attacks felt like
- What made the pain worse and what made it better
- What other symptoms (nausea, vomiting, sensitivity to sound and light, etc.) you experienced
- What potential triggers (food, hormones, weather, stress, etc.) you were exposed to 24 to 48 hours in advance of an attack
- What medications or treatments you took and how they worked

Your triggers can change throughout life. Always be on the lookout for new ones, and be open to the possibility that you may outgrow some.

The following list of triggers includes those that are most common. Not all migraine sufferers will be affected by these triggers. Finding what is specific to you and avoiding or managing your triggers is the key. The five most common migraine triggers are:

HORMONAL CYCLES OR CHANGES

- puberty
- menstruation
- birth control pills
- hormone replacement therapy
- perimenopause

CHANGES IN DAILY ROUTINE

- missing a meal
- sleeping more or less than usual

STRESS

- experiencing an episode of emotional stress
- resting after an emotionally stressful period

WEATHER AND ENVIRONMENT

- changes in barometric pressure
- cigarette smoke (first and secondhand)

DIETARY

- caffeine (coffee, tea, soft drinks) and, especially, caffeine withdrawal
- chocolate in any form
- fruits, especially citrus: oranges, lemons, limes, grapefruit, fermented dry fruits (raisins, figs, etc.), banana peel extract, red plums, papaya, and passion fruit
- beverages: beer, colored alcohol and wine (especially red, port, sherry, sweet white), dark rum, rye, brandy, and scotch
- dairy products: cultured dairy products such as sour cream and buttermilk; chocolate milk; acidophilus milk; aged cheese: Boursault, brick, Brie, Colby, Camembert, cheddar, Gouda, Gruyère, mozzarella, Parmesan, Emmentaler, provolone, Romano, Roquefort, and Stilton
- food additives: aspartame—NutraSweet; MSG: Accent, ajinomoto, Chinese seasoning, flavorings (including natural), glutacyl, glutavene, gourmet powder, hydrolyzed plant protein, hydrolyzed vegetable protein, kombo extract, mei-jing, RL-50, subu, vestin, wei-jing, and Zest
- nuts: peanuts
- seeds: sesame, sunflower, and pumpkin
- beans and vegetables: beans (lima, Italian, pole, broad, fava, navy, pinto, garbanzo, lentils, string), snow peas, chili peppers, pickles, olives, onions, garlic, peas, and tomatoes
- miscellaneous: brewer's yeast
- meat, fish, poultry: chicken and beef organ meats (liver and kidney), salted or dried fish (caplin, herring, cod), fermented sausage, bacon and processed meats (sodium nitrate)

HINT: Always read the labels of prepared foods, as many of these products contain additives such as MSG that may trigger a migraine attack. For a more detailed discussion of how to manage dietary triggers, see pp. 17–21.

{ Managing Migraine }

After obtaining a diagnosis, you should take the following important steps in managing your migraine:

- Identify your triggers by keeping a diary (see p. 22.)
- Keep a record of your triggers, as they can change over your lifetime.
- Optimize physical health by maintaining a healthy diet, exercising, keeping a regular sleep regimen, and taking medications correctly.
- Optimize mental health, and learn ways to manage the stress in your life.
- Consult regularly with your physician regarding treatment options.
- Obtain up-to-date information from your physician. Other good sources of information include the New York Headache Center in New York City, the Migraine Action Association in Great Britain, and the web site of the Journal of the American Medical Association (JAMA), where you can access their migraine Information Center.

MEDICATION

When you discuss treatment options with your doctor, be aware that there are two basic types of migraine medication: symptomatic and preventive.

Symptomatic medications are taken to relieve the symptoms of an attack once it's in progress. These medications are usually more effective when they are taken in the early stages of the attack. The most common types of symptomatic medications that are available over the counter are acetylsalicylic acid (ASA), acetaminophen, and ibuprofen.

Many symptomatic medications are currently available with a prescription, including a class of drugs called triptans. Triptan medications are known to the medical community as 5-HT (serotonin) receptor agonists. These medications work on the mechanism of migraine and relieve symptoms associated with it, such as headache pain, nausea/vomiting, and sensitivity to light and sound. Triptan medications narrow (constrict) blood vessels in the head that expand (dilate) during a migraine attack. They are also thought to reduce the release of substances that cause blood vessels to become inflamed and to reduce transmission of pain impulses to the brain.

Preventive medications are taken daily to prevent or reduce the frequency of migraine attacks. Unlike symptomatic medications, they are not pain relievers. They work for many sufferers by correcting the underlying imbalances within the body that are believed to cause migraine. All preventive medications should be taken exactly as prescribed. They take time to start working, so before their effectiveness is evaluated, they should be given at least two months to start to work.

Preventive drugs include beta-blockers, calcium channel blockers, antidepressants, monoamine-oxidase inhibitors (MAOIs), antiserotonin agents, anti-inflammatory agents, and anticonvulsants.

If you are interested in knowing more about any of these medications, consult your physician.

COMPLEMENTARY THERAPIES

A broad range of treatments for migraine do not fall within the category of conventional medicine. These include:

- biobehavioral treatment, such as biofeedback
- relaxation therapy and cognitive-behavioral therapy
- bodywork or manipulation, such as chiropractic, massage, and acupuncture
- vitamin, mineral, or herbal therapies, such as riboflavin, magnesium, and feverfew

These therapies are considered "complementary," or "nonpharmacological," and for many play an important role in prevention and empowerment. (Many migraine sufferers often feel powerless over their disorder and become frustrated or angry at the lack of validation from medical professionals, family members, employers, and friends.) These approaches are particularly useful when conventional treatment is inadequate, not tolerated, or contraindicated. The appropriateness of using such therapies is based on availability, cost, and the motivation and commitment of the individual seeking treatment.

In seeking treatment, it is always important to get an initial diagnosis (see p. 10) and follow-up from a doctor. It is also important to return to a physician if there is a change in symptoms and before beginning new therapies. Beware of therapists who will not allow you to see anyone else at the same time or who tout costly "miracle cures." Ask practitioners about their qualifications and whether their area of specialty is regulated by a professional organization. Ask them about the theory behind their method, and talk to others who have undergone the same therapy.

Biofeedback allows you to learn to alter your physiological responses at will. Machines provide feedback about biological responses in the body, such as the contraction of scalp muscles and the circulation and temperature of the hands or temple area. This information is then translated into a display—an audio tone or visual representation—that is "fed back" to the patient.

Relaxation therapy develops long-term skills for the prevention of migraine. Different methods include muscle relaxation, breathing exercises, and directed imagery. Relaxation therapy is often combined with biofeedback.

Cognitive-behavioral therapy (CBT) helps migraine sufferers identify stressful circumstances and employ effective strategies for coping. Individuals identify and modify negative responses that may trigger or aggravate migraine. CBT may also help to limit the negative psychological consequences of chronic pain, such as depression and disability. Similarly, **hypnotherapy** reduces distressing sensory input, which can act as triggers or aggravators of migraine.

Chiropractic may relieve some migraine attacks. Too much or too little movement in the cervical or neck region can cause muscle spasms around the neck, that may lead to a migraine attack. Manipulation, exercise, and physical therapy improve motion and can alleviate pain.

Massage has sedative and invigorating effects, increases range of motion, improves muscle tone and stimulates the release of endorphins, the body's natural painkillers. By massaging trigger points at the top of the neck and the base of the skull, the tension associated with chronic pain may be relieved.

Acupuncture, a traditional Chinese medicine that uses needles to restore the balance of energy, is believed to block the transmission of pain and stimulate the release of endorphins.

Riboflavin,* or vitamin B_2 (400 mg), as well as magnesium* (400–600 mg) may help to reduce the frequency and severity of migraine if taken on a daily basis.

*Feverfew**, which comes from a plant belonging to the chrysanthemum family, may also help migraine sufferers. It is believed to work by reducing the release of a chemical closely linked to migraine; by inhibiting the secretion of prostaglandin, a substance involved in inflammation; and by stabilizing blood vessels, making them less sensitive to the release of chemicals. Brands of feverfew that bear Drug Identification Numbers (D.I.N.) are regulated for content and are considered more reliable sources for this product.

---

* Always check with your doctor if you are planning to use riboflavin, feverfew, or magnesium.

{ Managing Dietary Triggers }

While there is no known cure for migraines, understanding your triggers can help you take charge of your attacks so that you can get your life back. Not all people are affected by food triggers—but those who are affected will find that managing food triggers will ensure that you lead a life in which you are in control. Identifying and avoiding your food triggers will help give you back a measure of control over your life.

Arguably, one of the most modifiable factors in migraine management is diet. While controversy remains around the relationship between the frequency and severity of migraines and the consumption of certain foods and substances, such as additives and preservatives, contained in foods, there is little doubt that diet may play a significant role in triggering, or initiating, migraine. Adjusting your diet, not restricting it, will give you greater control over your attacks. While ensuring that you are consuming an adequate amount of nutrients, it will help you manage your migraine attacks and stay healthy, whether you experience these headaches frequently or intermittently.

A substantial number of migraine sufferers experience an attack shortly after (or within 24 to 48 hours of) consuming a particular food or combination of foods. As mentioned above, identifying your food triggers and then avoiding them in your diet is an important step in migraine management and in your taking back control. In this section, we will discuss food triggers and how to identify them; migraines and MSG; and how to track your food triggers by keeping a trigger diary.

The information in the following pages should help you to recognize the foods, as well as the chemicals and additives contained in foods, that may trigger your migraines. Then turn to the recipe section for meal planning suggestions that will have you eating delicious foods that should not trigger an attack. You will soon recognize that you are not at the mercy of your migraines, and that you have, at your fingertips and in your pantry, an arsenal with which to fight them.

It is important to note that the actual foods you eat are not necessarily the only triggers to your migraines. That is, they are usually collaborating with some of your other dietary habits, such as skipping meals, fasting, or delaying meals. Moreover, dietary triggers may also be interacting with other triggers, as discussed on p. 12–13—environmental, stress, medication-related, or hormonal.

{ Food Trigger or Food Allergy? }

A food trigger is not a food allergy. A food allergy is an immune system response to a protein contained in food. While some researchers believe that food allergies do cause headaches, most believe that they in themselves play no role, but that the substances contained within some foods trigger the headache by changing the body's neurochemical balance. For example, they alter the balance of the neurotransmitter serotonin (a kind of chemical messenger), or they narrow and then expand the blood vessels in the brain. It is important to note that since food allergies do not appear to cause migraines, allergy testing won't get you any further ahead in identifying your dietary triggers.

{ Anatomy of a Food Trigger }

You eat a hot dog for lunch or go to your favorite Chinese restaurant for dinner, and within 24 hours you suffer a debilitating migraine attack. Why does this happen? According to the *Canadian Medical Association Journal*, "[the] ingestion of foods containing nitrites, aspartame, or monosodium glutamate, and the cumulative effect of eating foods with a high content of neurotransmitter precursors such as tyramine, tyrosine and phenylalanine, are associated with the precipitation of migraine headache." Hot dogs and other smoked or preserved meats such as luncheon meats, ham, bacon, and sausage contain nitrites; and Chinese food is notorious for containing the flavor enhancer monosodium glutamate (see p. 20). Both of these substances are implicated in the triggering of migraine attacks. They cause neurological disturbances that make the blood vessels in the brain swell, which further causes them to press on the surrounding nerves, and this may trigger an attack.

Many foods that initiate migraine attacks contain substances called vasoactive amines that affect the body's blood vessels, especially those that supply blood to the brain. Vasoactive amines widen or narrow the blood vessels in the brain, and this is responsible for the pain of the migraine headache. Food sources include any items that have been fermented (for example, ripened cheeses). These foods contain a substance known as tyramine. Tyramine can also be found in red organ meats such as beef and chicken liver and any pickled products.

Another amine implicated in migraines is phenylethlamine, a food source of which is chocolate in any form. Citrus fruits and their juices contain another headache-producing amine, synephrine.

Common sources of amine-containing foods include: fruit (avocado, banana, citrus fruits, pineapple, red-skinned fruits); vegetables (spinach, eggplant, the skin of potatoes and tomatoes); beverages (dark alcoholic drinks, tea); dairy products (ripened cheeses, buttermilk, yogurt, sour cream); herbs and spices; and cured, pickled, or marinated products. It is important to note that the amount of amine may be very slight and, in many cases, is not enough to trigger an attack.

{ The Migraine Sufferer's Pantry }

A variety of foods and food additives are known to trigger migraine attacks (see p. 13 for a list of the common dietary triggers), but it is important to note that not all of these foods act as triggers to everyone. A person who is sensitive to one food may, in fact, be able to eat it in small quantities if they have managed to control other triggers. As mentioned earlier, food triggers often do not act alone, but in collaboration with other triggers (see p. 11).

PROFILES OF THE USUAL SUSPECTS

Caffeine: Caffeine—or caffeine withdrawal—is often a trigger. In some cases, the ingestion of excessive amounts as part of a medication may be the culprit. Coffee and tea are common trigger foods, but remember that caffeine is also present in chocolate and soft drinks.

Chocolate: The more concentrated the chocolate, the more likely it is to trigger a migraine. Unsweetened and bittersweet chocolate, for example, are the most concentrated. Some people can consume milk chocolate or white chocolate in modest amounts and not risk suffering a migraine attack.

So, what's a chocoholic to do? Turn to the recipe section, and try Carob Chip Cookies (p. 154) or No-Bake Carob-Oatmeal Macaroons (p. 155). These delectable "chocolate" treats will make even the most hardened chocoholic's mouth water.

Fruit: The most common triggers in this category are citrus fruits (lemons, limes, oranges, and grapefruit). Some people can eat small quantities of these fruits and not suffer a migraine attack. Other food triggers in this category include papaya, mangoes, kiwi, pineapple, plums, avocado, and dried fruits that contain preservatives (for example, raisins, figs and dates.) These foods also contain vasoactive amines, that, as mentioned earlier, affect the blood vessels that supply blood to the brain.

Try the Wild Cherry Tabbouleh (p. 110) or the Roasted Pears with Mint Anglaise (p. 136) for some fruity delights.

Alcohol: Alcoholic beverages can dilate blood vessels in the brain and trigger migraine attacks. Red wine and other "colored" alcoholic beverages, such as dark rum, brandy, sherry, port, and scotch, are more common culprits in triggering attacks; the yeast contained in beer is also often implicated. Some migraine sufferers can tolerate white wine and other light-colored alcoholic drinks (vodka, for example) taken in modest amounts. It is important to remember that alcohol might negatively interact with medication you are taking for migraine as well as dehydrate you.

If you enjoy cooking with red wine and need a substitute for this potential food trigger, use vodka or white wine instead. Try the Phyllo-Wrapped Chicken with Mushrooms and Spinach in Citron Vodka Sauce (p. 74) or the Scallops with White Wine and Tarragon Sauce (p. 96).

For a soothing, nonalcoholic drink with medicinal qualities, try the Migraine Mellower (p. 148).

Dairy products: Cultured or fermented dairy products can be powerful triggers for some. Sources include yogurt and sour cream, chocolate milk, buttermilk, cultured butter, acidophilus milk and aged cheeses such as Boursault, brick, Brie, Camembert, cheddar, Gouda, Gruyère, mozzarella, Parmesan, Emmentaler, provolone, Romano, Roquefort, and Stilton. If you want to use cheese in a recipe, try unaged or mild cheeses, such as cottage cheese, goat cheese, or farmer cheese, and yogurt made from skim milk. Eggs are also a safe food choice. Also note that it is safe to drink 1% homogenized milk, 2%, or skim.

If you find yourself yearning for cheese, try the delicious Warmed Goat Cheese Salad with Grilled Vegetables (p. 48), the Toasted Creamy Goat Cheese with Onion Confit (p. 50), or the marvelous Vegetable and Cheese Lasagna (p. 61).

Monosodium glutamate (MSG): This substance can be a powerful migraine trigger. Common sources include packaged foods, powdered or canned soups, bouillon cubes, frozen dinners, and snack foods. There are also a number of hidden sources of MSG. Indeed, even if we carefully read food labels and decide the ingredients are "safe," we are frequently unaware of the MSG that is hidden in some other substance that is listed. MSG often lurks in the guise of polysyllabic, indecipherable ingredients.

Here is a list of ingredients that always contain MSG:

Monosodium glutamate	Hydrolyzed protein
Sodium caseinate	Yeast extract
Yeast nutrient	Autolyzed yeast
Textured protein	Yeast food
Calcium caseinate	Hydrolyzed oat flour

Artificial sweeteners: These substances, especially aspartame (NutraSweet, Equal) have been found to trigger migraine attacks in some people. Aspartame is frequently used in diet soft drinks and in sugarless chewing gum. Other artificial sweeteners, such as cyclamate (Sugar Twin) and sucralose (Splenda), do not appear to trigger migraine attacks.

Nuts and seeds: If you are predisposed to migraines, peanuts (and peanut butter) and seeds such as sesame, sunflower, and pumpkin seeds can be a trigger. We include avocados in this category, although people usually think of them as a fruit.

Beans and vegetables: Onions and tomatoes (although these are considered by some to be a fruit) are often identified as migraine triggers. Other triggers in this category include chili peppers, beans (lima, Italian, pole, broad, fava, navy, pinto, garbanzo, string), snow peas, and lentils. Olives, pickles, and sauerkraut have also been identified as possible culprits.

Delight in the fragrance and flavors of Steamed Basmati Rice with Crisp Potatoes, Sumac, and Cumin (p. 109), Bulgur and Green Bean Salad with Herbed Vinaigrette (p. 111), or Charred Zucchini with Herbs, Garlic, and Ricotta (p. 106).

Breads and yeast-raised baked goods: These foods contain yeast, which may trigger a migraine attack. Commercially prepared breads appear to present less of a problem than their hot, fresh, homemade counterparts. Before eating your homemade bread, let it sit for a while to cool; this may reduce its effect as a migraine trigger.

Try the Irish Scones (p. 127) or the Corn Bread (p. 129) for delicious breads that will not trigger a migraine attack.

Meat, poultry, and fish: Fresh beef, poultry, and fish are not implicated as migraine triggers, but organ meats such as kidney and liver may trigger an attack. Also in this category are processed or smoked meats, which contain nitrites (hot dogs, luncheon meats, ham, bacon, and sausage), and smoked, salted, or pickled fish.

Sample the Curried Chicken with Peaches and Coconut (p. 69), the Roast Duck with Spiced Honey (p. 76), or the Yellowfin Tuna with Maple Mustard Sauce and Coriander Oil (p. 86) for some succulent entrées.

Miscellaneous: Although it is rare, some people report suffering migraine attacks after consuming products containing food colorings and dyes, for example those used in candies, powdered drinks, and gelatin desserts. Others report attacks after consuming vinegar as contained in ketchup, mayonnaise, and salad dressings.

{ Don't Skip Meals }

If you are predisposed to migraines, don't skip meals—especially breakfast! A low blood sugar level caused by skipping meals or from other dietary practices such as irregular mealtimes or diets often trigger attacks. Skipping breakfast is an especially dangerous practice if you're a migraine sufferer; blood sugar levels are particularly low in the morning, and skipping breakfast can therefore trigger a headache later in the day. Turn to the recipe section, and let yourself be tempted by the Big Loonie Pancakes (p. 131) or the Apple Pancakes (p. 132.)

To keep your blood sugar levels stable during the day, eat a number of small meals at regular intervals, rather than two or three large meals. Consume these meals no more than four or five hours apart. Refer to the recipe section for snacks and meals that will keep your blood sugar levels from dipping too low. Sample the Yeast-Free Pretzels (p. 29) or the Herbed Pita Chips (p. 30) for a migraine-free dietary pick-me-up.

{ Tracking the Culprits: Your Food Trigger Diary }

Once you've examined the contents of your pantry and refrigerator and thought carefully about your food consumption patterns and all your triggers, you're well on the way to identifying the foods and beverages that may be responsible for triggering your migraine attacks. A diary in which you diligently track all the foods you eat each day will help you further identify the items to steer clear of.

Keeping a diary will help you determine your "trigger threshold"—the number of triggers you can be exposed to before experiencing an attack. For example, you may drink a cup of coffee and not end up in the grips of a migraine; but you may find that drinking a second cup, skipping a meal, and being overtired or overstressed will push you over the threshold, and you will experience a migraine attack.

In your diary, record:

- the food (or beverage) you consumed (include alcoholic beverages and those containing caffeine)
- the amount you consumed
- the time you consumed it (it may take your body 24 to 48 hours to react to a trigger)

Also record any headaches you experience, and note:

- date
- time of day

- location of head pain (behind the eyes; squeezing your head like a band; pounding on either side of your head; at the top of your head, radiating down the sides)
- duration
- frequency
- severity
- other symptoms (vomiting, nausea, sensitivity to light and sound)

You should also document other triggers such as weather, stress, hormonal fluctuations, and so on. As mentioned earlier, food triggers often work with other trigger accomplices.

TESTING YOUR TRIGGERS

As a pattern emerges, you may notice a correlation between your consumption of a food or beverage and the incidence and severity of your migraine attacks. Add these to your food triggers list, and avoid eating them; find delicious substitutes in the recipe section of this book.

Avoid the triggers identified in your diary, then reintroduce each of your "forbidden" foods. If you find you experience no symptoms when the food is not included in your diet, but the symptoms reappear when the food is reintroduced, it may be one of those triggering your migraine attack.

Documenting the foods and beverages you consume is not a complicated task and is well worth the effort in helping you get your life back. To obtain a copy of a migraine diary, contact an association near you. (See pp. 169–172 for a complete list of resources.)

CHECKLIST FOR AVOIDING MIGRAINES

1. Know your food triggers. Keep a list of them at hand, perhaps on the refrigerator door, where you can see them each time you're tempted to reach for that chocolate ice cream or a hunk of cheddar cheese.
2. Document the foods you eat each day in a migraine diary in order to identify the substances that may be initiating your attacks.
3. Note all your triggers, including your sleep patterns, changes in weather, hormonal fluctuations, and the incidence of stressful events.
4. Read food labels when you're shopping to make sure trigger ingredients are not contained in the items you are about to purchase. And be aware of hidden food triggers.
5. Enjoy the delectable, mouthwatering, migraine-free recipes in this book.

{ The Last Word . . . }

It is a challenge living comfortably with migraine; in fact, the idea that one can live comfortably with these often debilitating headaches may appear to be an absurd impossibility. However, by controlling the modifiable factors in your daily life, managing your triggers, and discussing treatment options with your doctor, you can regain control of your life.

You may wonder how on earth you're going to find anything to eat or how you're ever going to plan a meal, since everything you enjoy seems to be a potential trigger. The answer lies in some of the suggestions made in this section and in the recipe portion of this book. Use the recipes in the following pages to prepare mouthwatering dishes that are free of widely acknowledged food triggers. You will find recipes for appetizers and snacks, soups and salads, meatless main courses, meat and poultry, fish and seafood, vegetables and side dishes, breads, desserts and baked goods, and beverages. Plan your meals using these recipes, and you will enjoy eating wonderful foods with the knowledge that you are not setting yourself up for a migraine attack.

How to Use This Cookbook

The recipes found within these pages are delicious and nutritious. They range from easy-to-create to the more sophisticated.

Wherever possible, we have attempted to minimize the number of potential food triggers contained in the recipes, or we have suggested substitutions. To help you readily identify the recipes that are appropriate for you, we have included a trigger coding system for each recipe. It outlines the ten most common triggers and indicates the specific triggers that have been avoided or eliminated. For example, if a recipe contains no citrus fruit (lemon, lime, orange, or grapefruit), it is checked as being citrus-free.

Each recipe also contains a nutritional analysis, and all recipes are calculated per serving size, unless otherwise indicated. Where there is a choice, the nutritional analysis, is based on the smaller quantity and on the first ingredient. When ingredients are optional, they are not included in the analysis. Milk is calculated at 2% unless otherwise indicated.

In order to help you plan ahead, a ⊙ appears at the beginning of recipes with long preparation or cooking times.

Bon appétit!

Appetizers
AND Snacks

Yeast-Free Pretzels

{ MAKES ABOUT SIX 6" PRETZELS }

A wonderful alternative to bread pretzels for anyone who finds that yeast is a trigger.

NUTRIENTS PER SERVING
(1 PRETZEL):

Calories: 236
Protein: 7 grams
Fat: 8 grams
Carbohydrate: 34 grams

2	eggs, separated
¼ cup	softened margarine
2 cups	all-purpose flour
	Salt and pepper
	Milk
	Coarse salt

◆ In a small bowl, beat the egg whites until stiff, but not dry. In a separate bowl, beat the egg yolks until lemony.

◆ In a large bowl, with your hands or a spoon, work the egg yolks and margarine into the flour to form a dough-like mixture. Fold in the egg whites. Season with salt and pepper to taste. Roll out the dough, then slice and shape it into pretzels on a greased baking sheet. Brush with milk, and sprinkle with coarse salt. Bake at 350°F for about 10 minutes, turning over once. Serve the pretzels warm.

Herbed Pita Chips

These crispy and flavorful chips are ideal for a light snack.

THIS RECIPE IS *FREE* OF THE FOLLOWING TRIGGERS

Caffeine ✓

Chocolate ✓

Citrus fruits ✓

Red wine ✓

Aged cheese ✓

MSG & nitrates ✓

Aspartame ✓

Nuts ✓

Onions & garlic ✓

Yeast ✓

NUTRIENTS PER SERVING
(1 pita chip):

Calories: 30
Protein: trace
Fat: 2 grams
Carbohydrate: 3 grams

8	large pita pockets
1 cup	melted butter
1 tsp	each dried oregano, marjoram, basil, and parsley flakes

♦ Separate each pita pocket into two thin rounds. With scissors, cut the rounds into eighths. In a small bowl, combine the melted butter, oregano, marjoram, basil, and parsley; brush on the pita pieces. Place on a greased baking sheet, and bake at 300°F for 30 minutes.

Vegetable Platter
WITH Olive Oil Dip (Pinzimonio)

An Italian specialty, this healthy, easy-to-prepare appetizer consists simply of an assortment of fresh vegetables and extra virgin olive oil.

THIS RECIPE IS *FREE* OF THE FOLLOWING TRIGGERS

Caffeine ✓

Chocolate ✓

Citrus fruits ✓

Red wine ✓

Aged cheese ✓

MSG & nitrates

Aspartame ✓

Nuts ✓

Onions & garlic ✓

Yeast ✓

Fresh vegetables, such as carrots, cucumbers, red and yellow peppers, cherry tomatoes, fennel bulbs, and radishes, washed and cut up
Extra virgin olive oil
Salt
Crusty bread (optional)
Prosciutto, sliced paper thin (optional)

♦ Arrange the vegetables on a platter. (The quantity depends on how many people you are serving.) Drizzle olive oil onto individual plates, and season to taste with salt. The vegetables can be dipped into the olive oil. For additional flavor, serve with bread and prosciutto, although you'll want to avoid the latter if nitrates are a trigger for you.

{ **VARIATION:** Many vegetables can be served raw, but you may want to blanch some, such as green beans, sugar peas, and broccoli florets. }

Hummus

{ MAKES ABOUT 1 CUP }

A Middle Eastern specialty, hummus is ideal served with Herbed Pita Chips (see p. 30) or as a vegetable dip.

THIS RECIPE IS *FREE* OF THE FOLLOWING TRIGGERS

Caffeine ✓

Chocolate ✓

Citrus fruits

Red wine ✓

Aged cheese ✓

MSG & nitrates ✓

Aspartame ✓

Nuts ✓

Onions & garlic

Yeast ✓

NUTRIENTS PER SERVING
(1 Tbsp):

Calories: 59
Protein: 2 grams
Fat: 3 grams
Carbohydrate: 6 grams

1	14-oz can chickpeas
⅓ cup	hot water (approx.)
1	large lemon, juiced
2	cloves garlic
¼ cup	tahini
1 Tbsp	Virgin olive oil (approx.)
	Salt
	Chili powder

• Drain and thoroughly rinse the chickpeas. Puree in a food processor, gradually adding hot water to make a light consistency.

• Add the lemon juice, garlic, tahini, and olive oil; season with salt to taste. Process until well blended and smooth. Taste, and adjust the seasonings, if necessary.

• Transfer to a serving bowl, and garnish with chili powder.

{ **VARIATION:** Fresh chopped parsley and lightly toasted pine nuts can also be used as garnishes. }

Shiitake Pierogies WITH
Sweet Ginger Sauce

{ MAKES 6 SERVINGS }

These dainty vegetarian pierogies make an elegant and tasty appetizer. If MSG is a trigger, make sure you use a naturally brewed soy sauce or Homemade Soy Sauce (see p. 121).

THIS RECIPE IS *FREE* OF THE FOLLOWING TRIGGERS

Caffeine ✓

Chocolate ✓

Citrus fruits ✓

Red wine ✓

Aged cheese ✓

MSG & nitrates ✓

Aspartame ✓

Nuts ✓

Onions & garlic

Yeast ✓

NUTRIENTS PER SERVING:
Calories: 53
Protein: 1 gram
Fat: 1 gram
Carbohydrate: 10 grams

MAKE AHEAD: Shiitake Pierogies can be prepared up to a day ahead and stored in an airtight container in the refrigerator. Cook pierogies just prior to serving. The sauce can be prepared a day or two in advance, stored in the refrigerator, and heated prior to serving.

PIEROGIES

1 cup	mashed potatoes (cold leftovers are perfect)
1 cup	shiitake mushrooms, finely chopped (stems removed)
1	clove garlic, minced
½ tsp	fresh coriander leaves, finely chopped
1 pkg	oriental dumpling wrappers (available at oriental food stores; they're round and white)

SWEET GINGER SAUCE

2 tsp	soy sauce (naturally brewed or Homemade, p. 121)
1 tsp	cornstarch
½ cup	chicken or vegetable stock (see pp. 117–118)
1 tsp	minced ginger
2 tsp	granulated sugar
1 tsp	butter

• In a large bowl, mix the mashed potatoes with the mushrooms, garlic, and coriander. Place 1 tablespoon of the mixture on each dumpling wrapper, and wet the rim with water. Close and press together to seal. Boil or shallow-fry dumplings on high heat for about 3 minutes, or until cooked through. Set aside.

• To make the Sweet Ginger Sauce: Combine the soy sauce and cornstarch. Add it to the remaining ingredients in a saucepan. Bring to a boil; simmer until thickened.

• Serve Shiitake Pierogies in a pool of sauce, with sauce poured over them, or tossed with sauce.

Shrimp Rissoles

{ MAKES 6 SERVINGS }

These scrumptious appetizers—delicate morsels of shrimp inside a lightly fried golden crust—will keep your guests coming back for more. If lemon juice is a trigger for you, consider using finely chopped lemon grass instead.

THIS RECIPE IS *FREE* OF THE FOLLOWING TRIGGERS

Caffeine ✓

Chocolate ✓

Citrus fruits

Red wine ✓

Aged cheese ✓

MSG & nitrates ✓

Aspartame ✓

Nuts ✓

Onions & garlic

Yeast

NUTRIENTS PER SERVING:
Calories: 742
Protein: 18 grams
Fat: 38 grams
Carbohydrate: 82 grams

MAKE AHEAD: The shrimp filling can be prepared up to 2 days ahead and stored in the refrigerator. The rissoles can be assembled a day ahead, refrigerated, and cooked just before serving.

FILLING

2 Tbsp	olive oil
1	onion, chopped
2	cloves garlic, chopped
1 cup	baby shrimp, cleaned
1 cup	water
4	eggs
1 cup	milk
2 Tbsp	cake flour
2 Tbsp	cornstarch
	Salt and pepper
	Lemon juice, to taste
2 Tbsp	chopped parsley
Pinch	nutmeg

DOUGH

2 cups	water
2 cups	milk
⅔ cup	vegetable shortening
¼ cup	butter
Pinch	salt
	Pepper
2⅔ cups	all-purpose flour
⅔ cup	cake flour
⅔ cup	cornstarch
¼ cup	fine bread crumbs

To make the filling:

- In a medium saucepan, heat the olive oil over medium heat. Add the onion and garlic; cook until the onions are golden. Add the shrimp, and cook for 1 minute. Add the water, stirring until the mixture comes to a boil.

- Meanwhile, in a bowl, mix together 2 of the eggs, the milk, cake flour, and cornstarch. Add to the mixture in the saucepan.

- Add salt and pepper and lemon juice to taste. Add the parsley and nutmeg, and bring to a boil. Remove from the heat, and let the mixture cool.

To make the dough:

- In a large pot, combine the water, milk, shortening, butter, salt, and pepper to taste. Bring the mixture to a boil. Add the all-purpose flour, cake flour, and cornstarch; mix gradually until pasty. Remove from the heat.

- With a rolling pin on a floured surface, roll out the dough until it's ⅛″ thick all across. Cut into 3″ circles using a round cookie cutter. Place a spoonful of filling in the center of each circle. Fold over to form a half-moon shape and seal the dough.

- Brush the stuffed pastry with the two remaining beaten eggs, and toss the rissoles in the bread crumbs.

- Deep fry the rissoles (the oil must be at least 325°F) until golden. Let cool, and serve on a platter lined with lettuce leaves.

Grilled Gravlax WITH Mustard Dill Sauce

{ MAKES 4 SERVINGS }

The sweetly pungent dill sauce goes well with gravlax. Some mustards contain MSG, so watch for this potential trigger. The same amount of dry mustard can often be used instead.

NUTRIENTS PER SERVING:
Calories: 416
Protein: 21 grams
Fat: 36 grams
Carbohydrates: 2 grams

1 lb	gravlax, cut into 8 slices
	Extra virgin olive oil

MUSTARD DILL SAUCE

1 tsp	dry mustard powder
2 Tbsp	water
2 Tbsp	grainy Dijon mustard
1	egg yolk
1 tsp	granulated sugar
½ cup	vegetable oil
2 Tbsp	chopped fresh dill
	Dill sprigs

◆ To make the Mustard Dill Sauce: In a small bowl, dissolve the dry mustard powder in the water. Add the Dijon mustard, egg yolk, and sugar. Gradually whisk in the vegetable oil; add the dill.

◆ Lightly coat the gravlax with the extra virgin olive oil. Place on a preheated grill. Grill for 1 to 2 minutes per side, or until lightly seared.

◆ Place 2 slices of gravlax on individual salad plates; spoon some mustard sauce around the gravlax. Garnish with a sprig of fresh dill.

Soups AND Salads

Cream OF Mushroom Soup

{ MAKES 4 SERVINGS }

An earthy and satisfying beginning to a fall or winter meal. The recipe calls for a small amount of onion, but this ingredient can be omitted if it is a trigger for you.

THIS RECIPE IS *FREE* OF THE FOLLOWING TRIGGERS

Caffeine ✓

Chocolate ✓

Citrus fruits ✓

Red wine ✓

Aged cheese ✓

MSG & nitrates ✓

Aspartame ✓

Nuts ✓

Onions & garlic

Yeast ✓

NUTRIENTS PER SERVING:
Calories: 148
Protein: 6 grams
Fat: 8 grams
Carbohydrate: 13 grams

2 Tbsp	butter
1 tsp	chopped onion
1 cup	chopped mushrooms
3 Tbsp	all-purpose flour
1 tsp	salt
Pinch	pepper
2 cups	Chicken Stock (see p. 118)
2 cups	milk

◆ In a saucepan, melt the butter over medium heat; sauté the onion and mushrooms. Blend in the flour, and add the salt and pepper. Stir in Chicken Stock and milk. Heat until steaming, and serve immediately.

Cream of Spinach Soup

This soup is rich but light and tastes as fresh as spinach itself.

THIS RECIPE IS *FREE* OF THE FOLLOWING TRIGGERS

Caffeine ✓

Chocolate ✓

Citrus fruits ✓

Red wine ✓

Aged cheese ✓

MSG & nitrates ✓

Aspartame ✓

Nuts ✓

Onions & garlic

Yeast ✓

NUTRIENTS PER SERVING:
Calories: 112
Protein: 4 grams
Fat: 8 grams
Carbohydrate: 6 grams

4 cups	Chicken Stock (see p. 118)
2–3 cups	fresh spinach, chopped
1 slice	onion (omit if onion is trigger)
1 cup	10% cream (approx.)
	Salt and pepper
	Fresh parsley

- In a large saucepan, simmer Chicken Stock, spinach, and onion (if using) for about 10 minutes.

- In a blender, process the stock mixture until smooth. Return the mixture to saucepan, and heat. Add cream until the soup is the desired consistency. Add salt and pepper to taste. Serve garnished with chopped fresh parsley.

Pumpkin Bisque

{ MAKES 8 SERVINGS }

This smooth, full-flavored soup is a perfect make-ahead first course for an autumn dinner party. It also freezes well and can be reheated in the microwave.

THIS RECIPE IS *FREE* OF THE FOLLOWING TRIGGERS

Caffeine ✓

Chocolate ✓

Citrus fruits ✓

Red wine ✓

Aged cheese ✓

MSG & nitrates ✓

Aspartame ✓

Nuts ✓

Onions & garlic ✓

Yeast ✓

NUTRIENTS PER SERVING:
Calories: 108
Protein: 3 grams
Fat: 4 grams
Carbohydrate: 15 grams

2 Tbsp	butter
2	leeks (white part), thinly sliced
½ cup	each diced carrot and parsnip
5 cups	Chicken Stock (see p. 118)
2½ cups	pumpkin puree
1 tsp	dried thyme
½ tsp	salt
¼ tsp	pepper
Pinch	hot pepper flakes (optional)
½ cup	milk
2 Tbsp	snipped chives

- In a large saucepan, melt the butter over low heat. Add the leeks, carrots, and parsnips, and cook until softened, about 10 minutes.

- Stir in Chicken Stock, pumpkin puree, thyme, salt, pepper, and hot pepper flakes (if using).

- Bring to a boil, reduce the heat, cover, and simmer for 10 minutes, or until the vegetables are very soft.

- In a blender or food processor, puree in batches until smooth. Return to the saucepan. Stir in the milk; heat gently until hot (do not boil). Taste, and adjust seasoning. Serve sprinkled with chives.

Vichyssoise

This potato and leek soup is best served very cold. The potatoes provide a rich thickness, and the leeks lend a delicate flavor. If onions are a trigger, you might want to skip this recipe, because leeks and chives are in the same family of vegetables.

THIS RECIPE IS *FREE* OF THE FOLLOWING TRIGGERS

Caffeine ✓

Chocolate ✓

Citrus fruits ✓

Red wine ✓

Aged cheese ✓

MSG & nitrates ✓

Aspartame ✓

Nuts ✓

Onions & garlic

Yeast ✓

NUTRIENTS PER SERVING:
Calories: 259
Protein: 6 grams
Fat: 7 grams
Carbohydrate: 43 grams

1 Tbsp	butter
4	leeks, finely sliced
1	large onion, finely sliced
4	medium potatoes, peeled and diced
2 cups	Chicken Stock (see p. 118)
	Salt and pepper
½ cup	cream
	Chives or parsley

- In a saucepan, melt the butter over medium heat. Cook the leeks and onion until transparent (do not brown). Add the diced potatoes and Chicken Stock. Season with salt and pepper to taste. Cook slowly for about 30 minutes, or until the potatoes are tender.

- In a blender or food processor, puree until smooth.

- Refrigerate, covered, until cold, for at least 2 hours. Stir in the cream.

- Adjust the seasoning, if necessary, and ladle the soup into chilled bowls. Sprinkle with chives or chopped parsley before serving.

Curried Winter Vegetable Soup

{ MAKES 6 TO 8 SERVINGS }

This hearty soup can be adapted to meet specific dietary needs. For a little variety, add some chopped kale or leftover lettuce, and serve with toasted French bread. It's great served with warm biscuits (see Healthy Biscuits on p. 126).

1½ Tbsp	butter
1 tsp	each cumin, curry, rosemary, pepper, and sage
4–6	cloves garlic, minced
1	large leek, chopped
4 cups	Chicken or Vegetable Stock (see pp. 117–118)
1 cup	water
1	medium rutabaga, peeled and cubed
1 cup	split lentils (red and/or yellow)
2	medium sweet potatoes, peeled and diced
1	medium waxy potato, peeled and diced
2	medium carrots, peeled and sliced
1	medium parsnip, peeled and sliced
¼ cup	coconut milk (or regular milk if desired)
2 Tbsp	finely chopped cilantro or parsley

THIS RECIPE IS *FREE* OF THE FOLLOWING TRIGGERS

Caffeine ✓

Chocolate ✓

Citrus fruits ✓

Red wine ✓

Aged cheese ✓

MSG & nitrates ✓

Aspartame ✓

Nuts ✓

Onions & garlic ✓

Yeast ✓

NUTRIENTS PER SERVING
(when serving 6):

Calories
Protein g
Fat g
Carbohydrates g

◆ In a large stockpot, melt the butter. Stir in the cumin, curry, rosemary, pepper, and sage. Add the garlic and leek. Cook over low heat for 2 to 5 minutes, or until the leek is tender. Add the stock, water, rutabaga, and lentils. Bring to a boil slowly; reduce the heat, cover, and simmer for 10 minutes. Add the potatoes, carrots, and parsnip.

◆ Simmer, covered, for 25 to 40 minutes, or until the potatoes, carrots, and parsnips are tender. Remove from the heat; allow to cool slightly until all bubbling has stopped. Mash with a potato masher until the consistency is partly chunky. Stir in the coconut milk or regular milk and the cilantro or parsley. Heat briefly to rewarm, and serve.

{ **VARIATIONS:** Any vegetable can easily be added or substituted in this recipe. Cooked meat can also be added. Barley can be used instead of the lentils, but more cooking time should be allowed. }

Easy Fish Chowder

{ MAKES ABOUT 4 SERVINGS }

Serve this nutritious chowder with crackers or crusty bread.

THIS RECIPE IS *FREE* OF THE FOLLOWING TRIGGERS

Caffeine ✓

Chocolate ✓

Citrus fruits ✓

Red wine ✓

Aged cheese ✓

MSG & nitrates ✓

Aspartame ✓

Nuts ✓

Onions & garlic ✓

Yeast ✓

NUTRIENTS PER SERVING:
Calories: 392
Protein: 23 grams
Fat: 16 grams
Carbohydrate: 39 grams

2 Tbsp	butter
4	medium potatoes, diced
1 cup	thinly sliced celery
1 cup	grated carrot
1 tsp	rosemary
	Salt and pepper
½ lb	fish fillets (cod, haddock, or any firm white fish) or 1 can (5 oz) baby clams (with juice)
2 cups	whole evaporated milk

- In a large saucepan, melt the butter over medium heat. Lightly sauté the potatoes, celery, and carrot. Cover with water (or clam juice, if using). Add the rosemary and salt and pepper to taste. Simmer until tender.

- Add the fish, cut into pieces, and simmer until the fish flakes easily when tested with fork. Stir in the milk, and heat through without boiling. Just before serving, add salt and pepper to taste.

Roasted Potato Salad

{ MAKES 4 TO 6 SERVINGS }

A fresh and satisfying alternative to your mom's potato salad. Serve with a loaf of fresh crusty bread.

NUTRIENTS PER SERVING
(when serving 6):

Calories: 234

Protein: 4 grams

Fat: 10 grams

Carbohydrate: 32 grams

1	whole garlic head
1 Tbsp	olive oil +additonal for drizzling
	Salt and pepper
2 lbs	potatoes, scrubbed and cut into chunks
1	red pepper
⅓ cup	chopped red onion (approx.)

BALSAMIC VINAIGRETTE

¼ cup	olive oil or canola oil
2 Tbsp	balsamic vinegar or cider vinegar (if using cider, add 2 Tbsp brown sugar)
1 tsp	Dijon mustard (or the same amount of dry mustard if MSG is a trigger)
1 tsp	fresh thyme
Pinch	each cayenne, salt, and pepper

◆ Cut ½ inch off the garlic head, and place the garlic in a small baking dish. Drizzle with olive oil, and season with salt and pepper. Cover with aluminum foil. Bake at 300°F for 1½ hours, or until tender when squeezed. Let cool.

◆ In a roasting pan in a 425°F oven, heat 1 tablespoon olive oil until hot. Add the potatoes; toss to coat. Roast for 35 minutes or until soft and golden, turning often.

◆ To make the vinaigrette: In a small bowl, whisk together all the ingredients.

◆ Squeeze the roasted garlic pulp into a serving bowl. Add the potatoes, red pepper, onion, and vinaigrette. Toss. Adjust seasoning. Serve warm or at room temperature.

Grated Root Vegetable Salad
WITH Roasted Apple Dressing

{ MAKES 4 SERVINGS }

The unusual apple dressing gives this salad an exceptional flavor.

THIS RECIPE IS *FREE* OF THE FOLLOWING TRIGGERS

Caffeine ✓

Chocolate ✓

Citrus fruits ✓

Red wine ✓

Aged cheese ✓

MSG & nitrates ✓

Aspartame ✓

Nuts ✓

Onions & garlic ✓

Yeast ✓

NUTRIENTS PER SERVING:
Calories: 174
Protein: 2 grams
Fat: 6 grams
Carbohydrate: 28 grams

MAKE AHEAD: The dressing can be prepared earlier in the day and refrigerated.

2	Granny Smith apples, peeled and cored
	Olive oil
	Sea salt (optional)
2	medium red beets, peeled
2	parsnips, peeled
1	carrot, peeled
1	celery root, peeled
1	head lettuce

To make the dressing:

♦ Peel and core the apples, and arrange them neatly in a lightly oiled skillet.

♦ Season with sea salt, if desired, and cook over medium-high heat, turning occasionally, until the apples are tender and golden (do not let burn).

♦ Transfer the apples to a food processor, and process at high speed. Gradually pour in olive oil until the dressing is creamy.

To make the salad:

♦ Grate the vegetables, keeping them separate and covered until ready for serving.

♦ Spread dressing on individual salad plates, and arrange small mounds of grated vegetables around the rim. Place lettuce leaves in the center of each plate. Drizzle with the remaining dressing.

{ **KITCHEN POINTER:** Shred the vegetables as thin as possible. }

Middle Eastern Salad

{ MAKES 2 SERVINGS }

This is a fantastic salad with refreshingly different tastes.

NUTRIENTS PER SERVING:

Calories: 251

Protein: 2 grams

Fat: 23 grams

Carbohydrate: 9 grams

½	cucumber, chopped
	Salt and pepper
¼ cup	extra virgin olive oil
1 Tbsp	lemon juice
1	clove garlic, minced
1	tomato, finely chopped
½	red pepper, chopped
¼ cup	thinly sliced scallion
2 Tbsp	finely chopped fresh parsley
3 Tbsp	finely chopped fresh mint
	Mint sprigs

- In a colander, sprinkle the cucumber with a pinch of salt. Let drain for 20 minutes, and pat dry.

- In a large bowl, whisk together the olive oil, lemon juice, garlic, and salt and pepper to taste. Stir in the tomato, red pepper, scallion, parsley, and mint. Add the cucumber. Toss to mix well. Garnish with mint sprigs, and serve with toasted pita or falafel.

Warmed Goat Cheese Salad
WITH Grilled Vegetables

{ MAKES 2 TO 4 SERVINGS }

This fanciful salad brings together a wonderful assortment of vegetables. The same amount of dry mustard can be used instead of Dijon if MSG is a trigger.

THIS RECIPE IS *FREE* OF THE FOLLOWING TRIGGERS

Caffeine ✓

Chocolate ✓

Citrus fruits ✓

Red wine ✓

Aged cheese ✓

MSG & nitrates

Aspartame ✓

Nuts ✓

Onions & garlic ✓

Yeast

NUTRIENTS PER SERVING
(when serving 2):

Calories: 184

Protein: 10 grams

Fat: 8 grams

Carbohydrate: 18 grams

MAKE AHEAD: The dressing can be made earlier in the day. It will keep for 1 week if stored in an airtight container in the refrigerator.

1	small green zucchini
2	small eggplants
1	small red or green pepper, seeds removed
1	small fennel bulb, top stems removed
4 oz	goat cheese
1	egg
2 Tbsp	water
½ cup	Italian-style bread crumbs
1 cup	baby organic mixed salad greens

SALAD DRESSING (OPTIONAL)

½ cup	raspberry vinegar
1 Tbsp	Dijon mustard
1 Tbsp	Italian-style herbs (basil, thyme, oregano, etc.)
¾ cup	extra virgin olive oil
	Salt and pepper

● Trim the ends off the zucchini and eggplants. Cut them diagonally lengthwise into even-sized pieces.

● Cut the pepper lengthwise into 1"-wide strips.

● Cut the fennel bulb into quarters, then cut each quarter in half. Blanch the fennel in boiling salted water for approximately 5 minutes. Set aside.

● Cut the goat cheese into even-sized pieces (see Kitchen Pointer below).

● Break the egg into a bowl; add the water, and whisk together.

● Dip pieces of goat cheese into the egg. Thoroughly cover each piece with bread crumbs, and set aside.

To make the dressing (optional):

- In a bowl, mix the vinegar, Dijon, and herbs; whisk vigorously while slowly adding the oil. Season with salt and pepper to taste.

To assemble the salad:

- Toss the vegetables with a little oil, and season with salt and pepper. Grill them over high heat or under a broiler, turning them over when they are slightly charred (approximately 2 minutes.)

- Meanwhile, pour the dressing over the salad greens, and toss to thoroughly coat.

- Place equal amounts of salad onto individual salad plates, and arrange the vegetables around the salad. Warm the goat cheese under the broiler for approximately 1 minute; place on top of the salad.

{ KITCHEN POINTER: Goat cheese is best cut with dental floss to avoid breakage. }

Toasted Creamy Goat Cheese
WITH Onion Confit

{ MAKES 6 SERVINGS }

Toasted on eggplant with onion confit, creamy goat cheese has a marvelous flavor.

THIS RECIPE IS *FREE* OF THE FOLLOWING TRIGGERS

Caffeine ✓

Chocolate ✓

Citrus fruits ✓

Red wine ✓

Aged cheese ✓

MSG & nitrates ✓

Aspartame ✓

Nuts ✓

Onions & garlic

Yeast ✓

NUTRIENTS PER SERVING:
Calories: 441
Protein: 12 grams
Fat: 41 grams
Carbohydrate: 6 grams

MAKE AHEAD: The onion confit can be prepared a day in advance or earlier in the day.

½ cup	olive oil
2	onions, finely sliced
3	cloves garlic, finely chopped
1	bay leaf
¼ cup	dry white wine (optional)
2 Tbsp	white wine vinegar
	Salt and pepper
¼ cup	vegetable oil
1 Tbsp	balsamic vinegar
2 sprigs	fresh rosemary, leaves only, chopped
2 sprigs	fresh thyme, leaves only, chopped
1	eggplant, sliced crosswise into rounds
12 oz	goat cheese, cut into 2-oz rounds
1¾ cup	mixed baby greens
¼ cup	vinaigrette (your choice)

- In a pan over medium-high heat, heat the olive oil. Cook the onions, half of the garlic, and the bay leaf until the onions are transparent. Add the white wine and vinegar. Continue cooking until the confit is reduced to half. Add salt and pepper to taste.

- In a small bowl, combine the vegetable oil, the remaining garlic, balsamic vinegar, rosemary, thyme, and salt and pepper to taste. Brush this mixture onto the eggplant slices, and let sit for 10 minutes. Grill the eggplant over high heat, turning when slightly charred (approximately 2 minutes).

- Divide the confit evenly among the slices of grilled eggplant, then place the rounds of goat cheese on top. Place the eggplant on a baking sheet, and broil under a preheated broiler until light golden in color.

- Place several pieces of eggplant on top of the greens, forming a tower shape on individual salad plates. Drizzle with vinaigrette, and serve.

Grilled Portobello Mushrooms
WITH Goat Cheese AND Arugula

{ MAKES 2 SERVINGS }

The fresh herbs add a wonderful bouquet of flavors to this salad.

**THIS RECIPE IS *FREE* OF THE
FOLLOWING TRIGGERS**

Caffeine ✓

Chocolate ✓

Citrus fruits ✓

Red wine ✓

Aged cheese ✓

MSG & nitrates ✓

Aspartame ✓

Nuts ✓

Onions & garlic

Yeast ✓

NUTRIENTS PER SERVING:
Calories: 255
Protein: 6 grams
Fat: 19 grams
Carbohydrate: 15 grams

4	pieces Portobello mushrooms, medium size
2 Tbsp	extra virgin olive oil
1 Tbsp	balsamic vinegar
½ tsp	chopped garlic
Pinch	salt
1 tsp	each chopped fresh rosemary, thyme, and chives
1	bunch arugula (rinsed with cold water)
¼ cup	goat cheese, crumbled
Pinch	cracked black pepper
4	leaves fresh basil, shredded

• Brush the mushrooms with half of the olive oil, and grill on a medium-hot grill, turning frequently. When the mushrooms begin to release their water, remove them from the grill and set aside to keep warm.

• In a mixing bowl, whisk together the remaining olive oil, vinegar, garlic, salt, and chopped herbs.

• Arrange the arugula on two plates. Toss the warm mushrooms in the vinaigrette, and place on top of the arugula. Crumble goat cheese on top, and garnish around the salad with the black pepper and basil leaves.

{ **KITCHEN POINTER:** If you want to make this salad but don't have access to a grill, sauté the mushrooms in a pan over medium heat. To save time, the vinaigrette ingredients may be added right into the pan when the mushrooms are cooked. }

Black Bean Salad WITH Bell Peppers

{ MAKES 6 TO 8 SERVINGS }

This unique salad has great flavor, texture, and appearance.

THIS RECIPE IS *FREE* OF THE FOLLOWING TRIGGERS

Caffeine ✓

Chocolate ✓

Citrus fruits

Red wine ✓

Aged cheese ✓

MSG & nitrates ✓

Aspartame ✓

Nuts ✓

Onions & garlic

Yeast ✓

NUTRIENTS PER SERVING
(when serving 8):

Calories: 308
Protein: 10 grams
Fat: 12 grams
Carbohydrate: 40 grams

MAKE AHEAD: The salad can be made 6 hours ahead; let stand at room temperature. The vinaigrette can be made a day ahead. Before using, let itstand at room temperature.

VINAIGRETTE

½ cup	water
4 oz	raisins, chopped
½ cup	fresh lime juice
6 Tbsp	extra virgin olive oil
2 Tbsp	dried oregano
4 tsp	honey
4 tsp	each ground cumin and coriander
	Salt and pepper

SALAD

2	19-oz cans black beans, drained and rinsed
½ cup	each chopped red pepper, yellow pepper, green pepper, red onion, and fresh parsley

◆ To make the vinaigrette: In a heavy saucepan, boil the water and raisins for about 2 minutes. Remove from heat, cover, and let stand for about an hour to soften.

◆ Transfer the raisin mixture to a food processor. Add the lime juice, olive oil, oregano, honey, cumin, and coriander; process until smooth. Season to taste with salt and pepper.

◆ To make the salad: In a large bowl, toss the beans, peppers, onion, and parsley. Add enough dressing to coat. Season with salt and pepper to taste.

{ **VARIATION:** A combination of different types of beans (black, red, pinto) can be used for variety. }

Curried Chicken AND
Rice Salad WITH Almonds

{ MAKES 4 SERVINGS }

This flavorful dish is perfect served cold as a salad, but it can also be served hot as a main course. Worcestershire sauce sometimes contains MSG, so be aware of this potential trigger.

THIS RECIPE IS *FREE* OF THE FOLLOWING TRIGGERS

Caffeine ✓

Chocolate ✓

Citrus fruits ✓

Red wine ✓

Aged cheese ✓

MSG & nitrates

Aspartame ✓

Nuts

Onions & garlic

Yeast ✓

NUTRIENTS PER SERVING:
Calories: 722
Protein: 25 grams
Fat: 26 grams
Carbohydrate: 97 grams

2 cups	basmati rice
1½ cups	cooked chicken (skinless, boneless breasts)
2 Tbsp	olive oil
2 Tbsp	plain low-fat yogurt
1 Tbsp	curry powder
1 Tbsp	light soy sauce (naturally brewed or Homemade, see p. 121)
2 tsp	wine vinegar
1 tsp	celery seed
1 tsp	honey
1 tsp	Worcestershire sauce
½ tsp	garlic powder
½ tsp	pepper + additional to taste
1½ cups	diced red, yellow, or orange pepper
1 cup	slivered almonds
½ cup	diced celery
¼ cup	diced green onion
	Salt

- Cook the rice according to package instructions. Set aside.

- Dice the chicken. In a nonstick pan, lightly sauté the chicken with the olive oil, yogurt, curry powder, soy sauce, wine vinegar, celery seed, honey, Worcestershire sauce, garlic powder, and pepper until cooked through.

- Add the rice and the remaining ingredients. Cover, and simmer for about 5 minutes, or until the vegetables are tender. Season with salt and pepper to taste.

{ **VARIATION:** If serving the next day as a cold salad, add 1 tablespoon plain low-fat yogurt (to moisten) and 1/4 cup shredded carrot. Mix well. }

Warm Spinach Salad WITH Prawns

{ MAKES 2 SERVINGS }

A beautiful and elegant salad bursting with nutrition and flavor.

NUTRIENTS PER SERVING:
Calories: 217
Protein: 11 grams
Fat: 13 grams
Carbohydrate: 14 grams

1 bag	fresh spinach
2 Tbsp	olive oil
8	medium tiger prawns, cleaned
1	red pepper, julienned
2	Roma tomatoes, seeded and julienned
¼ cup	vinegar
	Salt and pepper

- Trim and wash the spinach. Pat dry.

- In a sauté pan over medium-high heat, heat the olive oil. Add the prawns, and cook until they turn red and firm.

- Add the red pepper and tomatoes; cook for 1 minute longer.

- Add the spinach and vinegar. Remove from heat, and gently toss. Season with salt and pepper to taste.

- Transfer to individual salad plates, and serve.

Meatless Main Courses

Roasted Wild Mushroom Veggie Burgers

{ MAKES 8 BURGERS }

Made with mushrooms and tofu, these are a delicious and nutritious alternative to regular beef patties. Worcestershire sauce sometimes contains MSG, so be aware of this potential trigger.

THIS RECIPE IS *FREE* OF THE FOLLOWING TRIGGERS

Caffeine ✓

Chocolate ✓

Citrus fruits ✓

Red wine ✓

Aged cheese ✓

MSG & nitrates

Aspartame ✓

Nuts ✓

Onions & garlic

Yeast

NUTRIENTS PER SERVING:
Calories: 205
Protein: 13 grams
Fat: 9 grams
Carbohydrate: 18 grams

2 Tbsp	olive oil
1	medium onion, chopped
Pinch	salt
1 cup	dry shiitake mushrooms, soaked in hot water until soft
2 cups	stemmed and chopped domestic, wild, or portobello mushrooms
16 oz	extra-firm tofu, mashed
¾ cup	quick-cooking oats
⅓ cup	toasted wheat germ
⅓ cup	bread crumbs
2 Tbsp	Worcestershire sauce
½ tsp	garlic powder

+ In a large nonstick skillet, heat the olive oil and sauté the onions and salt for about 5 minutes.

+ Stem the mushrooms. In a blender or food processor, mince all the mushrooms.

+ Add the mushrooms to the onions in the skillet, and cook for about 10 minutes, stirring occasionally.

+ Remove the mixture from the heat, and mix with the tofu. Add the remaining ingredients, and mix well. Measure out eight ½-cup portions. With wet hands, form them into patties.

+ Place the patties on a greased cookie sheet. Bake at 375°F for 25 minutes, turning once after 15 minutes. Just before serving, heat them in skillet or on a grill to heat through.

Chinese Noodle Salad with Roasted Eggplant

{ MAKES 4 TO 6 SERVINGS }

Here's an elegant dish that combines exciting flavors and textures. Mung beans can be found in Asian supermarkets.

THIS RECIPE IS *FREE* OF THE FOLLOWING TRIGGERS

Caffeine ✓

Chocolate ✓

Citrus fruits ✓

Red wine ✓

Aged cheese ✓

MSG & nitrates ✓

Aspartame ✓

Nuts ✓

Onions & garlic

Yeast ✓

NUTRIENTS PER SERVING:
Calories: 577
Protein: 16 grams
Fat: 25 grams
Carbohydrate: 72 grams

MARINADE AND NOODLES

½ cup	dark sesame oil
½ cup	soy sauce (naturally brewed or Homemade see p. 121)
3–4 Tbsp	sugar
3 Tbsp	balsamic vinegar
3 Tbsp	coriander, chopped
8–10	scallions, thinly sliced
1 Tbsp	red pepper oil
2½ tsp	salt
1	15-oz package chinese egg noddles (thinnest available) or linguine

EGGPLANT AND VEGETABLE GARNISHES

1 lb	firm, shiny Japanese eggplants
1 Tbsp	fresh ginger, peeled and minced
1	clove garlic, chopped
1 quart	water
1 tsp	salt
1 cup	blanched snow peas, string removed, cut into thin strips
½ lb	mung beans
3 Tbsp	sesame seeds (optional)
1	medium carrot, peeled and, julienned Coriander

To make the Marinade and Noodles:

◆ In a large bowl, combine all the ingredients except the noodles.

◆ Stir the marinade until the sugar dissolves.

◆ ◆ Bring a large pot of unsalted water to a boil. Gently pull apart the noodles, loosening and fluffing; add them to the boiling water. Cook the noodles until just tender, about 3 minutes. Drain, and place in a mixing bowl. Stir the marinade, pour half on the noodles, and toss. Set the remaining marinade aside.

To make the eggplant and vegetable garnishes:

◆ Preheat the oven to 400°F. In a baking dish, pierce the eggplants and bake until soft (about 20 minutes, depending on size), turning once. Let cool. Slice lengthwise, and peel the skin. Shred the eggplant into ¼" strips.

◆ Add the ginger and garlic to the reserved marinade. Add the eggplant strips to the mixture, turning them over several times. Set aside.

◆ Bring the water to a boil, and add the salt. Blanch the snow peas; rinse in cold water, and cut them into strips. Blanch the mung beans, and rinse. Lay them on a towel to dry.

◆ In a frying pan, roast the sesame seeds (if using) until lightly colored and fragrant.

◆ Toss the noodles with the eggplant strips and half of the sesame seeds.

◆ Mound the noodles on a platter. Distribute the carrots, snow peas, and mung beans over the noodles, and garnish with the remaining sesame seeds and coriander.

> **VARIATIONS:** Instead of sesame seeds, use roasted peanuts or cashews. Blanched asparagus tips can be used instead of eggplant. Long red or white radishes, thinly sliced and slivered, can also be included as a garnish.

Pasta Salad with Red Peppers and Artichokes

{ MAKES 4 TO 6 SERVINGS }

This colorful and tasty main course salad is ideal for a cold vegetarian lunch or a light supper.

NUTRIENTS PER SERVING
(when serving 6):

Calories: 463
Protein: 13 grams
Fat: 15 grams
Carbohydrate: 69 grams

1 lb	fusilli or penne
2	medium tomatoes, chopped
2	medium red or yellow peppers, chopped
1½ cups	black olives (optional)
¾ cup	marinated artichokes, drained and chopped
¼ cup	grated Parmesan cheese
⅓ cup	olive oil
1 Tbsp	red wine vinegar or cider vinegar
2 tsp	Dijon mustard (or the same amount of dry mustard if MSG is a trigger)
2 or 3	cloves garlic, peeled and minced
	Salt and pepper

- Bring a large pot of water to a boil. Add the pasta, and cook until just tender. Drain, and place in a large mixing bowl.

- Add the tomatoes, peppers, olives (if using), artichokes, and Parmesan cheese, and toss together.

- To make the dressing: In a small bowl, whisk together the olive oil, vinegar, mustard, and garlic.

- Toss the pasta with the dressing. Season with salt and pepper to taste, and serve.

Vegetable AND Cheese Lasagna

{ MAKES 2 SERVINGS }

A tasty dish that's easy when you use ready-made marinara sauce. If MSG is a trigger, make sure you choose the appropriate variety of marinara. This sauce may also contain onion, so read the label carefully.

THIS RECIPE IS *FREE* OF THE FOLLOWING TRIGGERS
Caffeine ✓
Chocolate ✓
Citrus fruits ✓
Red wine ✓
Aged cheese ✓
MSG & nitrates ✓
Aspartame ✓
Nuts ✓
Onions & garlic
Yeast

NUTRIENTS PER SERVING:
Calories: 529
Protein: 33 grams
Fat: 25 grams
Carbohydrate: 43 grams

1 cup	prepared marinara sauce
1 cup	coarsely chopped plum tomatoes
1	medium zucchini, thinly sliced
¼ cup	chopped fresh basil leaves or 1 tbsp dried
1 cup	ricotta cheese
⅔ cup	grated Parmesan cheese + additional to taste
	Salt and pepper
3	lasagna noodles

- In a heavy saucepan over medium heat, simmer the marinara sauce, tomatoes, zucchini, and basil for about 8 minutes, or until the zucchini is tender, stirring occasionally.

- In a bowl, mix the ricotta and ½ cup of the Parmesan. Season with salt and pepper to taste.

- In pot of boiling salted water, cook the lasagna noodles until just tender. Drain. Cut in half crosswise to make 6 pieces.

- Set aside 2 tablespoons of the sauce for topping. Place 2 noodle pieces in a greased 8″ square glass baking dish. Spread ¼ of the cheese mixture, then ¼ of the sauce over each noodle piece. Repeat. Finish with 2 noodle pieces, the reserved sauce, and the remaining Parmesan.

- Bake at 375°F, uncovered, for about 15 minutes, or until hot and bubbling. Serve with additional Parmesan cheese to taste.

{ **VARIATION:** You can make this lasagna with whatever vegetables you have on hand; for example, mushrooms, spinach, and onions could easily be substituted. }

Grilled Portobello Mushrooms
WITH Asparagus AND Herbed Polenta

{ MAKES 6 SERVINGS }

In this hearty dish, the polenta is herbed and eaten soft.

NUTRIENTS PER SERVING:

Calories: 372

Protein: 8 grams

Fat: 8 grams

Carbohydrate: 67 grams

MAKE AHEAD: The polenta can be prepared earlier and warmed just prior to serving.

6	medium portobello mushrooms
4 tsp	extra virgin olive oil
	Salt and freshly ground pepper
1	bunch asparagus, washed and peeled
1 lb	instant polenta
2 Tbsp	unsalted butter
1 Tbsp	each fresh rosemary, thyme, and parsley, chopped

- Clean the mushrooms, and brush with 3 teaspoons of the olive oil. Season with salt and pepper to taste.

- In a large skillet of boiling salted water, cook the asparagus for 2 to 3 minutes. Remove the asparagus, and refresh it by plunging it into a bowl of ice-cold water. Drain, and let dry by placing the asparagus on a pan or plate lined with paper towels.

- Grill the asparagus and mushrooms over medium heat for 2 to 4 minutes, or until just tender; watch carefully.

- In a large saucepan of boiling salted water, add the remaining olive oil and polenta. Cook for 6 minutes over medium heat.

- Remove the polenta from the heat, and stir in the butter and herbs until smooth.

- To serve, spoon the polenta onto a platter, and arrange the asparagus and mushrooms. Season with freshly ground pepper, if desired.

Stir-Fried Fresh Vegetables AND Tofu

{ MAKES 4 SERVINGS }

This stir-fry can be made with or without the tofu. Either way, the simple sauce adds an excellent flavor. Serve over rice for a complete meal.

THIS RECIPE IS *FREE* OF THE FOLLOWING TRIGGERS

Caffeine ✓

Chocolate ✓

Citrus fruits ✓

Red wine ✓

Aged cheese ✓

MSG & nitrates ✓

Aspartame ✓

Nuts ✓

Onions & garlic

Yeast ✓

NUTRIENTS PER SERVING:
Calories: 490
Protein: 18 grams
Fat: 30 grams
Carbohydrate: 32 grams

6 Tbsp	olive oil
8 oz	firm tofu, well drained, cut into ½" cubes
2 Tbsp	peeled and minced fresh ginger
3	cloves garlic, minced
1 lb	fresh shiitake mushrooms, stems trimmed, caps sliced
2 cups	broccoli florets
2	red peppers, cut into strips
2	bunches green onions, cut into 1" pieces
½ cup	dry white wine
¼ cup	soy sauce (naturally brewed or Homemade, see p. 121)
1 Tbsp	sesame oil
	Salt and pepper

• In a large nonstick skillet or wok, heat 3 tablespoons of the olive oil over high heat. Add the tofu, and stir gently for about 4 minutes, until it starts to brown around the edges. Transfer to a bowl.

• Add the remaining oil, ginger, and garlic to the skillet, and stir-fry for about 1 minute. Add the mushrooms, and stir-fry for about 5 minutes, or until tender around edges. Add the broccoli, red peppers, and green onions; stir-fry for about 3 minutes, or until just tender. Add the tofu to the skillet, and mix. Add the white wine, soy sauce, and sesame oil. Simmer for about 1 minute, or until heated through.

• Before serving, season with salt and pepper to taste.

Meat AND Poultry

Homestyle Chicken AND Rice Casserole

{ MAKES 4 TO 6 SERVINGS }

This is comfort food at its tastiest and easiest.

THIS RECIPE IS *FREE* OF THE FOLLOWING TRIGGERS

Caffeine ✓

Chocolate ✓

Citrus fruits ✓

Red wine ✓

Aged cheese ✓

MSG & nitrates

Aspartame ✓

Nuts ✓

Onions & garlic

Yeast ✓

NUTRIENTS PER SERVING
(when serving 6):

Calories: 389

Protein: 16 grams

Fat: 9 grams

Carbohydrate: 61 grams

2 cups	cooked, chopped chicken
2 cups	uncooked rice
2	10-oz cans cream of mushroom soup (without MSG) or homemade (see p. 39)
1 cup	water
5	green onions, chopped
3 tsp	curry powder
2 tsp	salt
1 tsp	sage
½ tsp	pepper

• In a large bowl, mix all the ingredients, stirring well. Pour into a 3-quart casserole dish. Bake at 325°F for 2 hours, or until the liquid is absorbed and the rice is tender.

{ **VARIATION:** Try adding ½ cup chopped broccoli before baking for something a little different. }

Simple Chicken Kiev

{ MAKES 4 SERVINGS }

This recipe turns a complicated old-world dish into a tasty and easy-to-prepare modern-day delight. Serve it with rice.

THIS RECIPE IS *FREE* OF THE FOLLOWING TRIGGERS

Caffeine ✓

Chocolate ✓

Citrus fruits ✓

Red wine ✓

Aged cheese ✓

MSG & nitrates ✓

Aspartame ✓

Nuts ✓

Onions & garlic

Yeast

NUTRIENTS PER SERVING:
Calories: 278
Protein: 32 grams
Fat: 10 grams
Carbohydrate: 15 grams

4	boneless, skinless chicken breasts
	Salt and pepper
4 tsp	margarine
4 tsp	chopped chives
½ tsp	tarragon
2	eggs
2 tsp	water
¼ cup	all-purpose flour
½ cup	dry bread crumbs

- Sprinkle each chicken breast with salt and pepper. Place 1 teaspoon of the margarine on each breast, and top with 1 teaspoon of the chives and a pinch of tarragon. Fold the chicken to enclose the filling completely, and secure with toothpicks.

- In a small bowl, beat the eggs and water. Coat the chicken with the flour, then dip it into the egg mixture. Coat with the bread crumbs. Place the chicken seam-side up in a greased baking pan.

- Bake at 400°F for 20 minutes, turning once, or until the juices run clear when the chicken is pierced with a fork.

Curried Chicken WITH Peaches AND Coconut

{ MAKES 4 TO 6 SERVINGS }

For a simple accompaniment, serve this chicken dish with basmati rice.

THIS RECIPE IS *FREE* OF THE FOLLOWING TRIGGERS

Caffeine ✓

Chocolate ✓

Citrus fruits ✓

Red wine ✓

Aged cheese ✓

MSG & nitrates ✓

Aspartame ✓

Nuts ✓

Onions & garlic

Yeast ✓

NUTRIENTS PER SERVING
(when serving 6):

Calories: 397
Protein: 33 grams
Fat: 25 grams
Carbohydrate: 10 grams

2 Tbsp	butter
1 Tbsp	oil
3½ lbs	frying chicken, cut into pieces
2 Tbsp	chopped onion (omit if a trigger)
1	small clove garlic, chopped (omit if a trigger)
1 cup	diced peaches, fresh or canned (drained if canned)
⅔ cup	Chicken Stock (see p. 118)
1½ tsp	curry powder
½ tsp	cumin
¼ tsp	brown sugar
	Salt and pepper
	Peach slices
	Shredded coconut

- In a large skillet, heat the butter and oil over medium-high heat. Add the chicken pieces; brown slowly on all sides. Remove from the skillet.

- Add the onion and garlic, and cook for 4 to 5 minutes, or until the onion is transparent. Add the diced peaches; cook, stirring, until the mixture is well combined, about 2 minutes.

- Meanwhile, combine the stock, curry powder, cumin, and brown sugar in a bowl. Add to the skillet, and heat for 5 minutes.

- Return the chicken to the skillet and season with salt and pepper to taste. Cover, and simmer until tender, about 25 to 30 minutes. Remove the chicken, and place it on a heated serving platter; keep warm.

- Add sliced peaches to the sauce. Cook just until glazed, pour the sauce over the chicken, and garnish with the coconut.

Japanese Glazed Chicken

{ MAKES 4 SERVINGS }

This delectable dish is perfect for an Asian-inspired meal. Serve it with rice and mixed vegetables.

NUTRIENTS PER SERVING:

Calories: 480

Protein: 36 grams

Fat: 8 grams

Carbohydrate: 66 grams

8	boneless, skinless chicken thighs
1	egg
1 cup	milk
1½ cups	all-purpose flour
½ cup	granulated sugar
½ cup	vinegar
3 Tbsp	water
3 Tbsp	soy sauce (naturally brewed or Homemade, see p. 121)
1 tsp	salt

- Trim the excess fat from the chicken. In a bowl, mix the egg and milk. Dip each chicken piece in the egg/milk mixture, and coat it in flour. In a frying pan over medium heat, brown the chicken lightly on both sides, approximately 2 to 3 minutes per side.

- Meanwhile, in a medium-size bowl, combine the remaining ingredients.

- When the chicken is browned, arrange it in a 13″×9″ pan (preferably glass), pour the soy mixture over the top. Bake at 350°F for 1 hour, basting the chicken with pan juices every 15 minutes.

Pasta with Chicken, Asparagus, and Sweet Red Pepper

{ MAKES 2 TO 4 SERVINGS }

The Dijon and rosemary give this pasta dish a beautifully mellow flavor.

THIS RECIPE IS *FREE* OF THE FOLLOWING TRIGGERS

Caffeine ✓

Chocolate ✓

Citrus fruits ✓

Red wine ✓

Aged cheese ✓

MSG & nitrates

Aspartame ✓

Nuts ✓

Onions & garlic

Yeast ✓

NUTRIENTS PER SERVING
(when serving 4):

Calories: 538
Protein: 22 grams
Fat: 34 grams
Carbohydrate: 36 grams

2 cups	bow tie (farfalle) pasta
2	boneless, skinless chicken breasts
1	bunch asparagus
1	sweet red pepper
3 Tbsp	olive oil
2 Tbsp	Dijon mustard (or the same amount of dry mustard if MSG is a trigger)
1 Tbsp	chopped garlic
1 Tbsp	chopped fresh rosemary
½ cup	dry white wine (optional)
1 cup	35% whipping cream
	Salt and pepper

• In a large pot of boiling salted water, cook the pasta until tender but firm, approximately 6 to 8 minutes. Drain, and set aside.

• Cut the chicken into bite-size pieces, and set aside.

• Wash and cut the asparagus into 1″ pieces, and set aside.

• Cut the red pepper in half; remove the seeds, and cut lengthwise into thin strips. Set aside.

• In a medium frying pan, heat the olive oil over medium heat. Add the chicken, and cook for approximately 5 minutes. Add the asparagus, and continue cooking for another 2 minutes. Add the mustard, garlic, rosemary, and red peppers, and cook for 1 minute.

• Add the wine (if using), and allow it to reduce by half. Add the whipping cream, and reduce until the mixture begins to thicken. Season to taste with salt and pepper.

• Add the pasta, and stir until thoroughly mixed and the pasta is reheated. Serve immediately.

Chicken Kabobs
WITH Homemade Barbecue Sauce

{ MAKES 10 SERVINGS }

The deep and mellow flavor of the barbecue sauce makes it the perfect accompaniment to grilled chicken. Many brands of mustard and ketchup contain MSG, so watch for these potential triggers.

THIS RECIPE IS *FREE* OF THE FOLLOWING TRIGGERS

Caffeine ✓

Chocolate ✓

Citrus fruits ✓

Red wine ✓

Aged cheese ✓

MSG & nitrates ✓

Aspartame ✓

Nuts ✓

Onions & garlic

Yeast ✓

NUTRIENTS PER SERVING:
Calories: 167
Protein: 28 grams
Fat: 3 grams
Carbohydrate: 7 grams

MAKE AHEAD: The barbecue sauce can be made 2 days in advance, while the kabobs can be prepared 1 day in advance. Store in the refrigerator until ready to grill.

BARBECUE SAUCE

6	cloves garlic, crushed
1	medium onion, chopped
1 cup	ketchup
¼ cup	water
¼ cup	maple syrup
3 Tbsp	Dijon mustard (or the same amount of dry mustard if MSG is a trigger)
3 Tbsp	balsamic vinegar
2 Tbsp	molasses
1 tsp	each chopped fresh thyme, rosemary, basil, marjoram, and oregano
1 tsp	ground cumin

KABOBS

10	boneless, skinless chicken breasts (each cut in half lengthwise, then cut in strips)
1	each red, yellow, and green pepper, each cut into 20 ½" square pieces

To make the barbecue sauce:
+ In a bowl, combine all the ingredients. Set aside.

To make the kabobs:
+ Marinate the chicken in 1 cup of the barbecue sauce overnight. Soak 20 bamboo skewers in water overnight.

+ Thread the chicken and peppers onto the skewers, alternating chicken with different-colored peppers. Make 20 kabobs, allowing 2 per person.

+ On a preheated barbecue, grill the kabobs for 3 to 5 minutes per side, or until the chicken is no longer pink inside. Baste with sauce as needed during grilling.

+ Serve on a bed of steamed rice.

Poached Chicken
WITH **Wild Rice** AND **Baby Vegetables**

{ MAKES 4 SERVINGS }

The rich and creamy sauce makes this dish elegant enough for company.

NUTRIENTS PER SERVING:

Calories: 603

Protein: 37 grams

Fat: 27 grams

Carbohydrate: 53 grams

* Wild rice must be soaked for at least 6 hours in fresh, cold water before cooking.

1 cup	mix of wild* and long grain rice
4 cups	Chicken Stock (see p. 118)
4	boneless, skinless chicken breasts
3	celery stalks, sliced into 1" sticks
2	parsnips, peeled and sliced into 1/4" rounds
1	carrot, peeled and sliced into 1/4" rounds
1	bunch Swiss chard, washed and coarsely chopped
1 cup	35% cream
	Salt and pepper
1	bunch Italian parsley, coarsely chopped

♦ In an ovenproof pot with a lid, cover the rice mixture with the stock to about 1 inch above the rice. Bake, covered, at 450°F for about 35 minutes. Remove, and let stand for 15 minutes.

♦ In a stewing pot, arrange the chicken and vegetables. Cover with the remaining stock, and bring to a boil over medium heat.

♦ Reduce the heat to maintain the simmer, and cook for about 10 minutes.

♦ Remove the chicken and vegetables from the stock, keep warm and covered until serving time. Bring the stock to a boil once more, and add the cream. Stir frequently until the sauce becomes thick enough to coat a spoon. Season with salt and pepper to taste.

♦ To serve, spoon the rice onto a serving dish or individual plates, creating a bed. Place the chicken and vegetables on top of the rice. Garnish with the parsley, and serve.

Phyllo-Wrapped Chicken WITH Mushrooms AND Spinach IN Citron Vodka Sauce

{ MAKES 4 SERVINGS }

Want to try something different? This classic recipe combines the delicate flavors of chicken, mushrooms, and spinach with the zesty taste of lemon. If lemon juice is a trigger, try using extra amounts of lemon grass (available at oriental markets and many supermarkets).

THIS RECIPE IS *FREE* OF THE FOLLOWING TRIGGERS

Caffeine ✓

Chocolate ✓

Citrus fruits ✓

Red wine ✓

Aged cheese ✓

MSG & nitrates ✓

Aspartame ✓

Nuts ✓

Onions & garlic

Yeast ✓

NUTRIENTS PER SERVING:
Calories: 531
Protein: 22 grams
Fat: 35 grams
Carbohydrate: 32 grams

MAKE AHEAD: Follow the recipe, and wrap the chicken in the phyllo earlier in the day; cover tightly with plastic wrap, and store in the refrigerator. Bake just before serving time.

1 pkg	fresh spinach, trimmed
2	boneless skinless chicken breasts, lightly pounded
1 cup	sliced button mushrooms
¼ cup	melted butter or oil + additional for brushing
1 cup	cooked rice
4 sheets	phyllo pastry

SAUCE

1 cup	35% cream
½ cup	Chicken Stock (see p. 118)
1 tsp	lemon juice
1 tsp	lemon grass, finely chopped (optional)
1 oz	citron vodka (optional)
	Salt

◆ Wash the spinach; shake off the excess water and place the spinach in a saucepan. With water clinging to the leaves, cook the spinach, uncovered, until wilted. Drain, squeeze the excess moisture from the spinach, and chop.

◆ In a large skillet, sauté the chicken breasts until they are seared on the outside. Remove, and let cool slightly.

◆ In the skillet, sauté the mushrooms in the butter or oil. Add the rice and chopped spinach to the mushrooms. Let cool slightly.

◆ Brush one phyllo sheet with butter or oil. Place a second sheet on top, and brush lightly with butter or oil. Fold in half.

◆ Divide the spinach mixture in two. Place in a pile on the phyllo. Place a chicken breast on top, and fold it together. Repeat with the other chicken breast.

- Bake at 400°F for about 15 to 20 minutes, or until the chicken is no longer pink inside and the pastry is golden brown.

- Meanwhile, in a saucepan, bring the cream, stock, lemon juice, and lemon grass to a boil; let simmer for a few minutes, until lightly thickened.

- Add the vodka to the sauce, if using.

- Season with salt to taste. (If lemon grass is unavailable, use basil, thyme, or a mixture of lemon zest and thyme.) To serve, place a generous amount of sauce on individual plates; place phyllo-wrapped chicken in the center of each plate.

Roast Duck WITH Spiced Honey

The succulent flavor of roast duck is combined with the sweet goodness of honey and spice in this elegant entrée. Perfect for entertaining!

THIS RECIPE IS *FREE* OF THE FOLLOWING TRIGGERS

Caffeine ✓

Chocolate ✓

Citrus fruits ✓

Red wine ✓

Aged cheese ✓

MSG & nitrates ✓

Aspartame ✓

Nuts ✓

Onions & garlic ✓

Yeast ✓

NUTRIENTS PER SERVING
(when serving 6):

Calories: 902

Protein: 48 grams

Fat: 70 grams

Carbohydrate: 20 grams

2	ducks (each 4 to 5 lb), cut in half lengthwise
	Salt and pepper
½ cup	honey
1 Tbsp	cumin
1 Tbsp	ground fennel seed

- Preheat the oven to 450°F.

- Place the duck halves skin-side down on a cutting board. Trim any excess fat to the edge of the skin. Generously season the inside and outside of the halves with salt and pepper.

- Place the duck halves, breast-side up, on a roasting rack set in a shallow baking pan. Roast in the preheated oven for 20 minutes. Reduce the heat to 375°F and continue roasting for another 20 minutes.

- Meanwhile, in a small bowl, mix the honey with the cumin and fennel seed to form a baste.

- Remove the duck from the oven, and baste with the honey mixture. Return the duck to the oven, and cook for an additional 20 minutes, or until the skin appears crisp.

{ **KITCHEN POINTER:** Cooking times may vary depending upon the size and weight of the duck. Check with your butcher to verify appropriate cooking times. }

Swedish Meatballs

{ MAKES 6 TO 8 SERVINGS }

This classic dish is a wonderful combination of spiced beef in a creamy sauce. Serve with rice or noodles, a crisp green salad, and crusty bread to mop up the sauce.

THIS RECIPE IS *FREE* OF THE FOLLOWING TRIGGERS

Caffeine ✓

Chocolate ✓

Citrus fruits ✓

Red wine ✓

Aged cheese ✓

MSG & nitrates ✓

Aspartame ✓

Nuts ✓

Onions & garlic

Yeast

NUTRIENTS PER SERVING
(when serving 8):

Calories: 564

Protein: 31 grams

Fat: 40 grams

Carbohydrate: 20 grams

1 cup	fine bread crumbs
2½ cups	milk
2 lbs	lean ground beef
2	eggs, lightly beaten
1½ tsp	salt
¼ tsp	pepper
1 tsp	nutmeg
½ cup	butter or margarine
¼ cup	all-purpose flour
3 cups	Beef Stock (see p. 118)
1½ cups	light cream

- In a large bowl, soften the bread crumbs in 1 cup of the milk. Add the beef, eggs, and seasonings; mix well. Shape into 1″ balls. In a large skillet, brown the meatballs in butter or margarine. Remove from the skillet, and set aside.

- In the same skillet, add the flour to the skillet drippings, and blend well. Gradually add the stock, the remaining milk, and the cream to the flour mixture, and cook over low heat, stirring constantly, for about 3 minutes.

- Add the meatballs to the sauce, and simmer for 10 to 15 minutes, or until heated through, stirring occasionally. Transfer to a covered dish, and serve.

Sweet AND Sour Pork Chops

{ MAKES 4 SERVINGS }

This tangy dish is delicious served with potatoes and spinach.

THIS RECIPE IS *FREE* OF THE FOLLOWING TRIGGERS

Caffeine ✓

Chocolate ✓

Citrus fruits ✓

Red wine ✓

Aged cheese ✓

MSG & nitrates

Aspartame ✓

Nuts ✓

Onions & garlic

Yeast ✓

NUTRIENTS PER SERVING:
Calories: 329
Protein: 22 grams
Fat: 9 grams
Carbohydrate: 40 grams

¾ cup	water
½ cup	brown sugar
½ cup	ketchup
½ cup	white vinegar
2 Tbsp	Worcestershire sauce
1 tsp	chili powder
4–6	pork chops
2	medium onions, sliced

♦ In a large bowl, mix the water, sugar, ketchup, vinegar, Worcestershire sauce, and chili powder.

♦ Place the pork chops in a roasting pan, and cover with the onions.

♦ Pour the sauce over the pork chops and onions. Cover, and cook at 300°F for about 1 to 1½ hours, or until the chops are tender.

Pork Tenderloin WITH Fresh Tomato Sauce

{ MAKES 4 SERVINGS }

These tender pieces of pork cook quickly and are a perfect accompaniment to the savory tomato-based sauce.

NUTRIENTS PER SERVING:

Calories: 680

Protein: 44 grams

Fat: 12 grams

Carbohydrate: 99 grams

2 Tbsp	olive oil
1 lb	pork tenderloin, cubed
½ cup	green pepper, coarsely chopped
1	clove garlic, chopped
1	celery stalk, coarsely chopped
2 cups	seeded and chopped tomatoes
½ tsp	each fresh thyme, oregano, and basil
	Salt and pepper
1 lb	fettuccine

+ In a large skillet over medium-high heat, heat the olive oil. Sauté the pork until brown. Remove the pork, and set aside. Keeping warm.

+ In the same skillet, cook the pepper, garlic, and celery until tender. Add the tomatoes, thyme, oregano, and basil, and simmer for 15 minutes longer.

+ Return the pork to the skillet, and cook for another 4 to 6 minutes. Season with salt and pepper to taste.

+ Meanwhile, in a large pot of boiling salted water, cook the pasta until al dente.

+ Drain the pasta, and serve with the pork mixture over top.

Honey-Roasted Lamb Tenderloin with Green Asparagus and Plantain Mash

{ MAKES 4 SERVINGS }

Delectable pieces of lamb are combined with a honey glaze and mixed with fresh green asparagus and the succulent flavor of roasted plantain.

THIS RECIPE IS *FREE* OF THE FOLLOWING TRIGGERS

Caffeine ✓
Chocolate ✓
Citrus fruits ✓
Red wine ✓
Aged cheese ✓
MSG & nitrates ✓
Aspartame ✓
Nuts ✓
Onions & garlic
Yeast ✓

NUTRIENTS PER SERVING:
Calories: 355
Protein: 18 grams
Fat: 15 grams
Carbohydrate: 37 grams

MAKE AHEAD: The plantain mash can be made earlier in the day and kept covered. Once cooled, put it in the refrigerator until needed. Reheat before serving.

2 Tbsp	honey
2 Tbsp	balsamic vinegar
4	lamb tenderloins
2	ripe plantains, skinned and chopped
1 tsp	olive oil
	Salt and pepper
¼ cup	Vegetable Stock (see p. 110)
1 cup	35% cream, reduced by half
2 Tbsp	vegetable oil
30	spears asparagus, cut about 4 inches

◆ In a small bowl, mix the honey and balsamic vinegar. Coat the lamb with this mixture, and marinate for 1 to 2 hours.

◆ Preheat the oven to 400°F. In a shallow roasting pan, toss the plantain with the olive oil and salt and pepper to taste. Cover with aluminum foil, and roast for 10 minutes.

◆ Add the vegetable stock to the plantain (reserve a bit of stock for mashing). Continue roasting for 5 to 7 more minutes, or until the plantain is very soft. Remove from the oven.

◆ In an electric mixer on medium-high speed, mix the plantain until mashed. Reduce the speed, and add the cream in a steady stream. Add any extra stock if the mash is too thick. Keep warm.

◆ Remove the lamb from the marinade; sprinkle with salt and pepper. In a nonstick pan, heat the vegetable oil over medium-high heat. Sear the lamb on all 4 sides, about 2 minutes per side.

- Remove the lamb, and keep warm. Drain most of the fat from the pan, then sear the asparagus for about 2 minutes, stirring occasionally, until bright green and tender.
- To serve, portion the lamb, asparagus, and plantain mash onto individual dinner plates.

{ **KITCHEN POINTER:** Lamb tenderloins are usually available frozen, 8 to a package. They are not large, so 2 per person makes a reasonable portion size. If you are preparing 8 tenderloins, remember to double the recipe amounts. }

Quick Lamb Patties

{ MAKES 2 SERVINGS }

Served with new potatoes and asparagus, these mint-flavored patties make a great meal. Chutney may contain citrus fruits or MSG, so watch for these potential triggers.

THIS RECIPE IS *FREE* OF THE FOLLOWING TRIGGERS

Caffeine ✓

Chocolate ✓

Citrus fruits

Red wine ✓

Aged cheese ✓

MSG & nitrates ✓

Aspartame ✓

Nuts ✓

Onions & garlic

Yeast ✓

NUTRIENTS PER SERVING:
Calories: 309
Protein: 27 grams
Fat: 21 grams
Carbohydrate: 3 grams

10 oz	ground lamb
1	green onion, finely chopped
1	clove garlic, finely chopped
2 Tbsp	minced fresh mint
	Salt and pepper
3 Tbsp	chutney

◆ Preheat the broiler. In a small bowl, combine the lamb with the onion, garlic, and mint. Season with salt and pepper to taste. Mix well.

◆ Shape the lamb mixture into 2 patties, each about 1″ thick.

◆ Under the broiler, broil the patties for about 4 minutes, or until brown. Turn them over, and broil for about 4 more minutes, or until they reach the desired doneness.

◆ Spread half of the chutney on each pattie. Continue broiling for about 1 minute more, or until the chutney begins to bubble. Transfer the patties to plates.

Fish AND Seafood

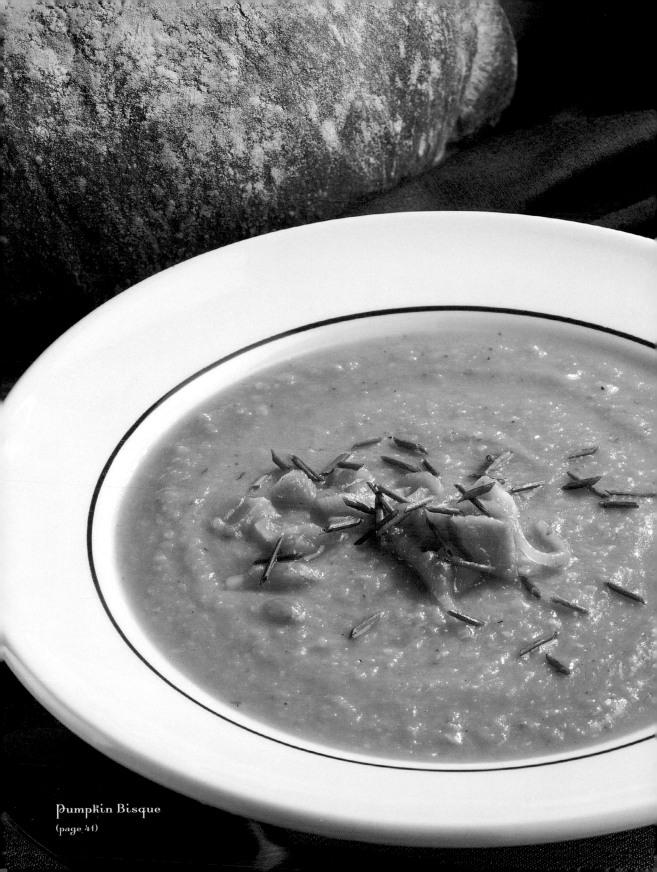

Pumpkin Bisque
(page 41)

Warmed Goat Cheese Salad
with Grilled Vegetables
(page 48)

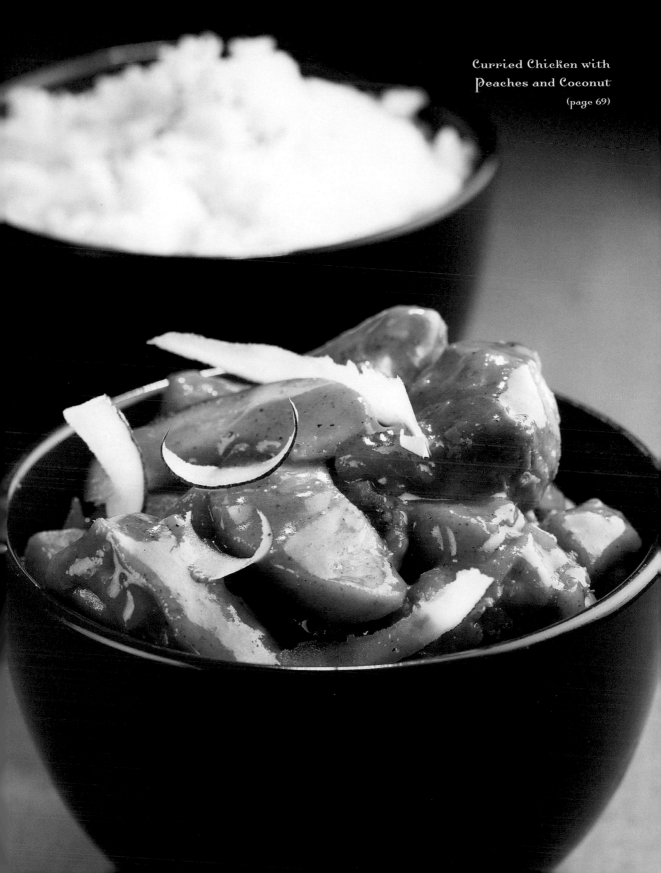

Curried Chicken with
Peaches and Coconut
(page 69)

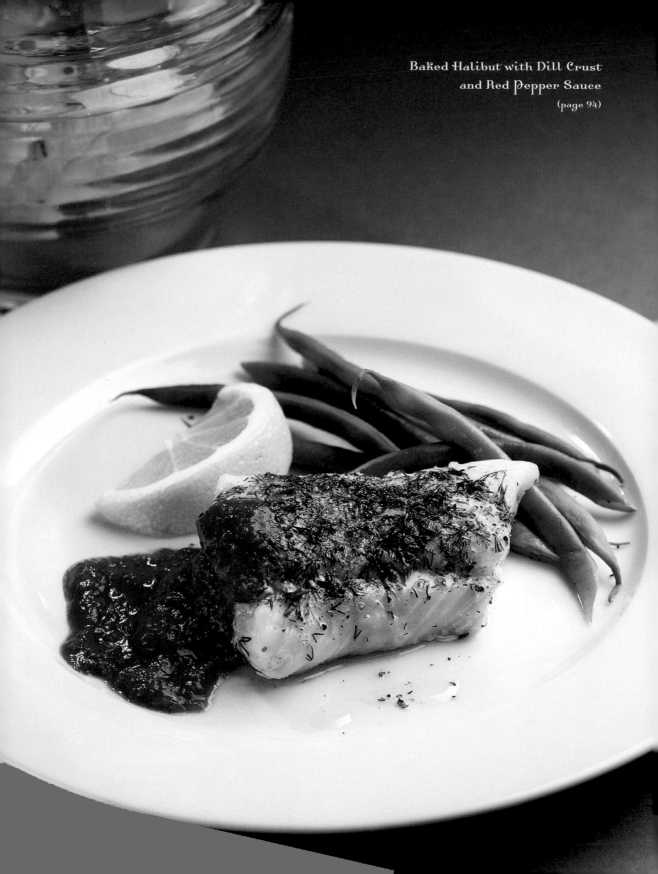

Baked Halibut with Dill Crust
and Red Pepper Sauce
(page 94)

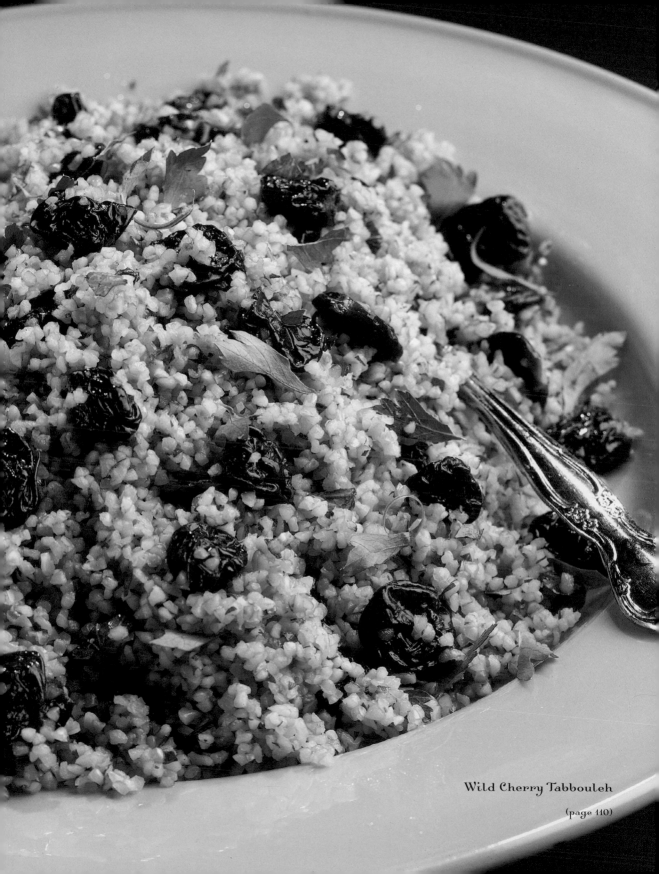

Wild Cherry Tabbouleh

(page 110)

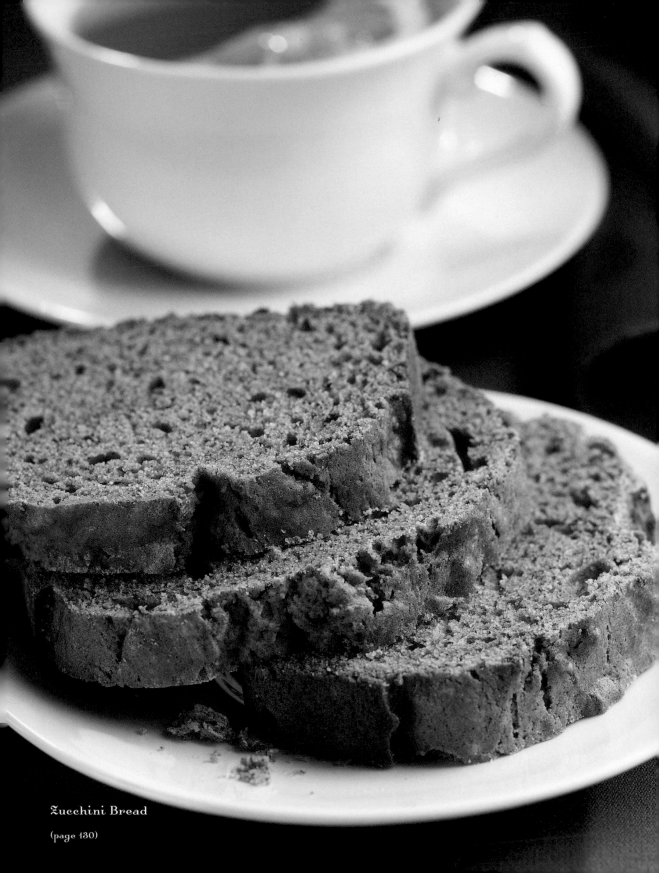

Zucchini Bread

(page 130)

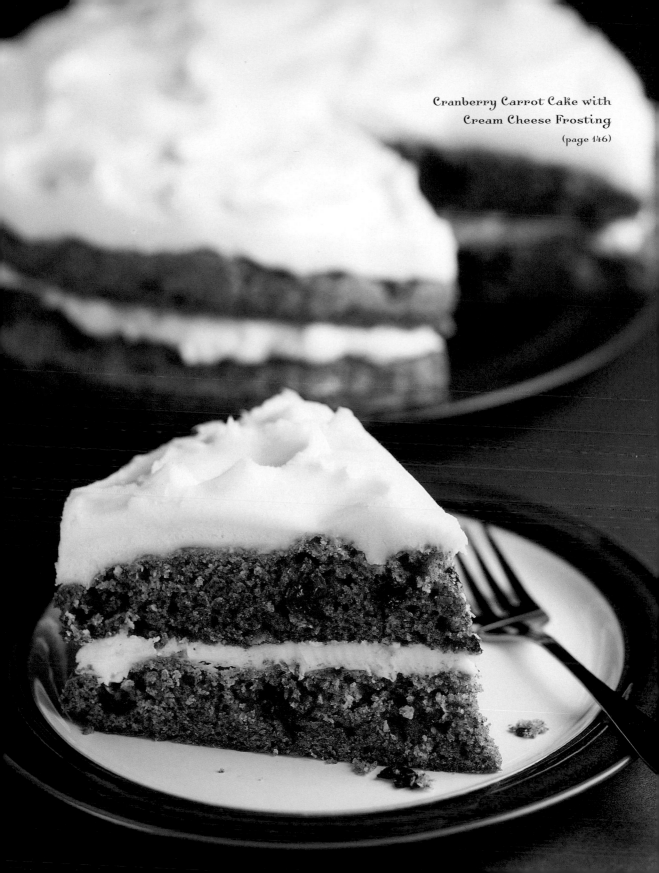

Cranberry Carrot Cake with
Cream Cheese Frosting
(page 146)

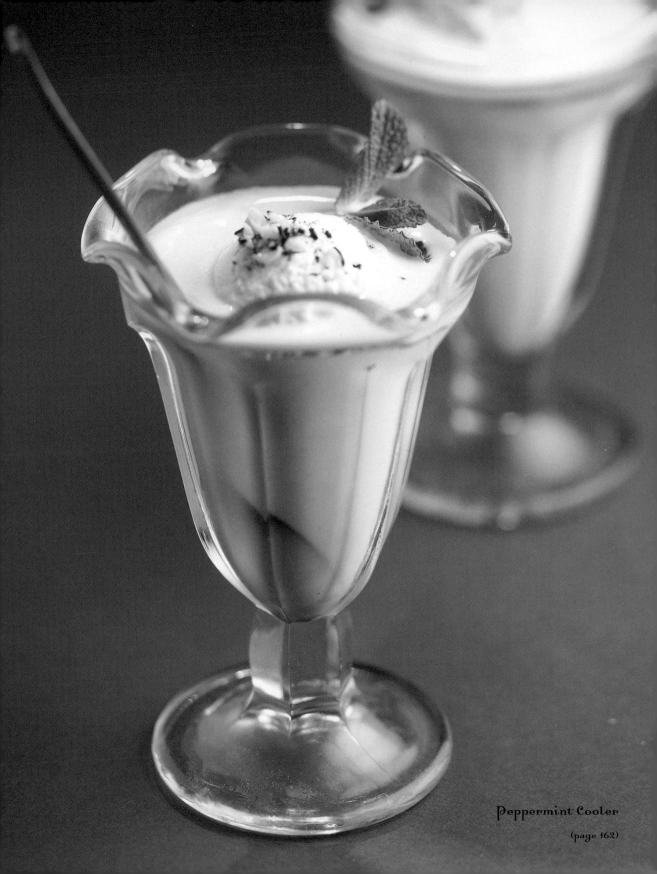

Peppermint Cooler

(page 162)

Easy Tuna Casserole

{ MAKES 2 TO 4 SERVINGS }

Here's a quick recipe using ingredients from the pantry and leftover cooked rice or pasta.

NUTRIENTS PER SERVING
(when serving 4):

Calories: 334
Protein: 18 grams
Fat: 10 grams
Carbohydrate: 43 grams

2 cups	cooked rice or pasta
1	6½ oz can water-packed tuna, drained
2 Tbsp	butter
1	stalk celery
2 Tbsp	all-purpose flour
2½ cups	milk
½ tsp	dillweed
	Salt and pepper
10	soda crackers, crushed

+ In a greased baking dish, combine the rice or pasta and tuna.

+ In a saucepan, melt the butter; cook the celery until transparent; stir in the flour until well combined.

+ Gradually add the milk, and stir until thickened. Add the dillweed and salt and pepper to taste.

+ Pour the sauce over the tuna mixture. Top with the crushed soda crackers.

+ Bake at 350°F for 15 minutes, or until bubbly around the edges.

Yellowfin Tuna
WITH Maple Mustard Sauce AND Coriander Oil

{ MAKES 2 TO 4 SERVINGS }

Do you want to test your culinary skills? This sophisticated recipe uses raw fish and requires that you build towers!

THIS RECIPE IS *FREE* OF THE FOLLOWING TRIGGERS

Caffeine ✓

Chocolate ✓

Citrus fruits

Red wine ✓

Aged cheese ✓

MSG & nitrates

Aspartame ✓

Nuts ✓

Onions & garlic

Yeast ✓

NUTRIENTS PER SERVING
(when serving 4):

Calories: 699
Protein: 30 grams
Fat: 55 grams
Carbohydrate: 21 grams

MAKE AHEAD: Towers can be made at least 1 hour ahead, covered with plastic wrap, and refrigerated. Yellowfin tuna can be replaced with salmon or salmon trout.

CORIANDER OIL

½ cup	chopped fresh coriander
2 Tbsp	chopped fresh parsley
½ cup	olive oil

MAPLE MUSTARD SAUCE

2 Tbsp	Dijon mustard (or the same amount of dry mustard if MSG is a trigger)
1 Tbsp	maple syrup
1 Tbsp	fresh lemon juice
2 tsp	sherry vinegar
¼ cup	grape seed or vegetable oil

YELLOWFIN TUNA

1	avocado, peeled, pitted, and diced
2 Tbsp	lemon juice
	Salt and pepper
1	mango, peeled, pitted, and diced
2 Tbsp	Coriander Oil
2	plum tomatoes, seeded and chopped
4 oz	yellowfin tuna, thinly diced
2 Tbsp	finely chopped onions
1 tsp	each mirin and tamari (optional)
3 Tbsp	chives, chopped
1 cup	shredded lettuce
4 tsp	yellow caviar (salmon roe)
2	6-oz yellowfin tuna (center cut)

To make the coriander oil:

◆ In a small pot of boiling salted water, blanch the coriander and parsley for 30 to 60 seconds, until bright green. Drain, plunge into cold water, and drain again. Dry in a salad spinner or with paper towels.

◆ In a blender, puree the coriander and parsley until smooth. In a steady stream, add the olive oil, and blend for 3 to 4 minutes. Pass it through a fine sieve or cheesecloth, and set aside.

To make the maple mustard emulsion:

◆ In a measuring cup or small bowl, whisk together the mustard, maple syrup, lemon juice, and sherry vinegar. Still whisking, drizzle in the grape seed or vegetable oil. Set aside.

To make the yellowfin tuna:

◆ In a small bowl, mix together the avocado, lemon juice, and salt and pepper to taste.

◆ In another small bowl, stir together the mango, 1 tablespoon of the coriander oil, and salt and pepper to taste.

◆ In another bowl, mix the tomatoes with the remaining tablespoon of coriander oil and salt and pepper to taste.

◆ Toss together the diced fish, onions, mirin, and tamari (if using), chives, and salt and pepper to taste.

To assemble:

◆ Using a 3″-round cookie cutter, build a tower in the center of a dinner plate by packing one quarter of the avocado mixture into the ring, followed by one quarter each of the mango, tomato, and fish mixtures. Pack lightly, and gently remove the ring.

◆ Top each tower with equal amounts of lettuce; Place a dollop of caviar on top of each.

◆ Arrange the fish pieces around the tower; drizzle the plate with the maple mustard.

{ **KITCHEN POINTER:** Mirin is a fermented rice wine with a trace of alcohol. Tamari is a gourmet soy sauce. Both are available at specialty food shops. }

Herb-Crusted Salmon Fillets

{ MAKES 4 SERVINGS }

The piquant-flavored crust of capers, horseradish, and fresh herbs pairs wonderfully with the mellow richness of roasted salmon. But horseradish is in the onion family, so watch for this potential trigger.

THIS RECIPE IS *FREE* OF THE FOLLOWING TRIGGERS

Caffeine ✓

Chocolate ✓

Citrus fruits ✓

Red wine ✓

Aged cheese ✓

MSG & nitrates ✓

Aspartame ✓

Nuts ✓

Onions & garlic

Yeast

NUTRIENTS PER SERVING:
Calories: 416
Protein: 37 grams
Fat: 20 grams
Carbohydrate: 22 grams

2 Tbsp	Italian parsley, leaves only
2 Tbsp	chopped chives
1 Tbsp	capers
1 Tbsp	fresh tarragon, leaves only
2 tsp	Dijon mustard (or the same amount of dry mustard if MSG is a trigger)
2 tsp	Worcestershire sauce (optional)
1 cup	fresh bread crumbs from white bread, finely crumbled
2 Tbsp	fresh horseradish, peeled and grated
	Salt and pepper
4	6-oz salmon fillets

- In a food processor, combine the parsley, chives, capers, tarragon, mustard, and Worcestershire sauce. Process for about 2 minutes, or until smooth.

- Transfer the puree to a mixing bowl. Add the bread crumbs, horseradish, and salt and pepper to taste.

- Mix until well combined. The mixture should be moist but should hold together when you squeeze it. If it is too wet, add more bread crumbs. If too dry, add water.

- Preheat the oven to 400°F. Place the fillets on lightly oiled baking sheet. Pack 1/4 cup of the mixture onto each fillet so that the surface is covered and the mix is about ½" thick. Bake for 15 minutes, or until the fish flakes easily when tested with a fork (reduce the baking time if you prefer salmon slightly rare.)

MAKE AHEAD: The bread crumb mixture can be prepared earlier in the day. If you would like a more generous crust, double the amounts for the bread crumb mixture.

Poached Salmon in Rosé

{ MAKES 10 SERVINGS }

Nothing could be more elegant than whole salmon poached in fragrant rosé and served with our Hollandaise Sauce.

THIS RECIPE IS *FREE* OF THE FOLLOWING TRIGGERS

Caffeine ✓

Chocolate ✓

Citrus fruits

Red wine

Aged cheese ✓

MSG & nitrates ✓

Aspartame ✓

Nuts ✓

Onions & garlic

Yeast ✓

NUTRIENTS PER SERVING
(with 2 Tbsp Hollandaise Sauce):

Calories: 330
Protein: 33 grams
Fat: 22 grams
Carbohydrate: trace

4 cups	water
¼ cup	chopped shallots
1	stalk celery with leaves, chopped
1	carrot, chopped
1	bunch fresh parsley
1 tsp	salt
2½ cups	rosé
1	whole, fresh salmon (4 to 5 lb)
2	lemons, cut in wedges
	Hollandaise Sauce (see p. 120)

◆ In a saucepan, combine the water, shallots, celery, carrot, four sprigs of parsley, and salt. Bring to a boil over medium-high heat; reduce the heat and simmer, uncovered, for 20 minutes.

◆ Pour this stock into a large roasting pan. Add the rosé.

◆ Wash the fish inside and out. Place it on a rack and into the pan. If the fish is not at least half covered by stock, add up to 1 cup extra water and more wine as necessary.

◆ Bring the stock to just under the boiling point so that the water appears to shiver rather than bubble. (If you cook fish faster than this, it will tend to fall apart.)

◆ Poach, covered, for 35 minutes, or just until the fish flakes easily when tested with a fork.

◆ Carefully lift the rack from the pan; remove any bits of vegetables. Place the fish on a platter; garnish with lemon wedges and the remaining parsley. Serve with Hollandaise Sauce (see p. 120.)

{ **VARIATION:** You can replace the salmon with red snapper. }

Salmon Wrapped in Rice Paper in a Yellow Pepper Sauce

{ MAKES 4 SERVINGS }

The fresh tastes of ginger and garlic blend beautifully with salmon. Serve this exotic dish with a fresh green salad. The commercially made sauces may contain MSG, so read the labels carefully.

THIS RECIPE IS *FREE* OF THE FOLLOWING TRIGGERS

Caffeine ✓

Chocolate ✓

Citrus fruits ✓

Red wine ✓

Aged cheese ✓

MSG & nitrates

Aspartame ✓

Nuts ✓

Onions & garlic

Yeast ✓

NUTRIENTS PER SERVING:

Calories: 319

Protein: 27 grams

Fat: 15 grams

Carbohydrate: 19 grams

1 lb	salmon fillets
4 pieces	rice paper
4 sprigs	each basil and coriander

MARINADE

2	cloves garlic, finely chopped
1 Tbsp	chopped coriander
2 tsp	fresh ginger, chopped
2 tsp	tamari sauce
1 tsp	each oyster sauce, mirin (optional), and sesame oil

SAUCE

1	clove garlic
1	large shallot, finely chopped
2	large yellow peppers, cut into small pieces
1½ cups	Fish or Vegetable Stock
1 tsp	Extra virgin olive oil
	Salt and pepper

To make the marinade:

- In a bowl, mix together all the ingredients.
- Pour it over the salmon fillets, and marinate for about 1 hour before assembling.

To make the sauce:

- In a saucepan over medium heat, sauté the garlic and shallot. Add the yellow peppers; deglaze with the stock.
- Cover, and simmer for 20 minutes, or until the peppers are tender.
- In a blender or food processor, or using a food mill, process the mixture until smooth. Add the oil, if necessary.
- Season with salt and pepper to taste. Set aside. The sauce should be reheated prior to serving.

To assemble:

- Remove the fish from the marinade. Dry gently, removing excess ingredients. Season with salt and pepper to taste.
- Dip each piece of rice paper in water until workable. Wrap each fillet in rice paper with sprigs of basil and coriander. Steam the fillets for 3 to 4 minutes in bamboo steamer set above a pot of rapidly boiling water, or in a fish steamer.
- Pour the reheated sauce on individual plates. Place the salmon on top of the sauce.

Grilled Salmon Steaks
WITH *Mango Strawberry Cilantro Chutney*

{ MAKES 2 SERVINGS }

The tanginess of strawberries and the sweetness of mango are the perfect combination for grilled salmon. Serve this dish with wild rice and ratatouille.

2	mangoes, semi-ripe
1 pint	strawberries
1	sweet red pepper, seeds removed
1	bunch cilantro or coriander
½ cup	water or white wine
2 Tbsp	honey
2 Tbsp	curry powder
1 Tbsp	cinnamon
2	salmon steaks (each 6 to 8 oz)
	Olive or vegetable oil
	Salt and pepper

THIS RECIPE IS *FREE* OF THE FOLLOWING TRIGGERS

Caffeine ✓
Chocolate ✓
Citrus fruits ✓
Red wine ✓
Aged cheese ✓
MSG & nitrates ✓
Aspartame ✓
Nuts ✓
Onions & garlic ✓
Yeast ✓

NUTRIENTS PER SERVING:
Calories: 342
Protein: 34 grams
Fat: 18 grams
Carbohydrate: 11 grams

MAKE AHEAD: The chutney can be prepared earlier in the day. Store it in the refrigerator, and bring it to room temperature prior to serving.

- Peel the mangoes, and separate the fruit from the pit. Dice into cubes, and set aside. Remove the stems from the strawberries, cut them into quarters, and set aside. Dice the red pepper into cubes, and set aside. Coarsely chop the cilantro, and set aside.

- In a small saucepan over medium heat, cook the red pepper for 1 minute.

- Add the mango, water or wine, honey, curry powder, and cinnamon. Reduce the heat to low, and simmer for approximately 10 minutes, or until the mixture resembles syrup.

- Add the strawberries and cilantro, and simmer for 2 minutes more.

- Rub the salmon steaks with oil, season with salt and pepper to taste, and grill or broil, turning them over every 3 minutes. Continue cooking until the fish is opaque or it reaches the desired doneness.

- Place the salmon on individual plates, and place a generous helping of mango chutney in the middle.

Pan-Seared River Trout
WITH Cucumber AND Baby Shrimp Salsa

{ MAKES 4 SERVINGS }

The fresh ingredients are what makes this dish so spectacular. Serve it with rice, potatoes, or noodles and your favorite vegetable.

THIS RECIPE IS *FREE* OF THE FOLLOWING TRIGGERS

Caffeine ✓

Chocolate ✓

Citrus fruits ✓

Red wine ✓

Aged cheese ✓

MSG & nitrates ✓

Aspartame ✓

Nuts ✓

Onions & garlic

Yeast ✓

NUTRIENTS PER SERVING:
Calories: 361
Protein: 42 grams
Fat: 17 grams
Carbohydrate: 10 grams

MAKE AHEAD: Prepare the salsa earlier in the day, and refrigerate it.

4	river or salmon trout, deboned and dressed

SALSA

1 cup	baby shrimp
1	red onion, diced
½	mango, sliced
½	sweet red pepper, diced
1	cucumber, ½ diced, ½ sliced
2 Tbsp	rice wine vinegar
2 Tbsp	olive oil + additional for sautéing
1 Tbsp	chopped fresh dill
	Salt and pepper

♦ To make the salsa: In a bowl, combine the shrimp, onion, mango, red pepper, diced cucumber, rice vinegar, olive oil, and dill. Mix well, and chill.

♦ Over medium heat, heat enough olive oil to generously cover the bottom of a 12-inch skillet. Season the trout with salt and pepper inside and out. Sauté each trout until golden, about 4 to 5 minutes per side.

♦ Transfer the trout to a warm plate, and decorate with the cucumber slices. Top with the salsa, and serve hot.

Baked Halibut WITH Dill Crust AND Red Pepper Sauce

{ MAKES 2 SERVINGS }

Sometimes it's the simplest ingredients that bring out the best in fish. Fresh dill, red pepper, garlic, and olive oil help to create a uniquely flavorful dish.

THIS RECIPE IS *FREE* OF THE FOLLOWING TRIGGERS

Caffeine ✓

Chocolate ✓

Citrus fruits ✓

Red wine ✓

Aged cheese ✓

MSG & nitrates ✓

Aspartame ✓

Nuts ✓

Onions & garlic

Yeast ✓

NUTRIENTS PER SERVING:
Calories: 224
Protein: 26 grams
Fat: 12 grams
Carbohydrate: 3 grams

½ lb	halibut fillets
1 tsp	olive oil
2 tsp	chopped fresh dill
	Salt and pepper

RED PEPPER SAUCE

1	red pepper, cored and seeded
1	clove garlic, chopped
1 Tbsp	olive oil
	Salt and pepper

- Place the fillets on a single piece of aluminum foil; drizzle with the olive oil. Top with the dill and salt and pepper to taste.

- Wrap the fillets tightly in the foil and place them on a baking sheet. Bake at 375°F for 10 to 12 minutes, or until the fish flakes easily when tested with a fork.

To make the sauce:

- Cut the pepper into large pieces. In a bowl, toss the pepper pieces with the garlic and oil.

- Roast in the oven until well colored.

- In a food processor, process until smooth. Pass through a sieve; season with salt and pepper to taste. Serve the sauce with the fillets.

Lemon Sole WITH Oranges AND Honey

{ MAKES 4 SERVINGS }

In this wonderful recipe, the delicate flavor of lemon sole is paired with the tanginess of oranges and the sublime sweetness of honey.

THIS RECIPE IS *FREE* OF THE FOLLOWING TRIGGERS

Caffeine ✓

Chocolate ✓

Citrus fruits

Red wine ✓

Aged cheese ✓

MSG & nitrates ✓

Aspartame ✓

Nuts ✓

Onions & garlic

Yeast ✓

NUTRIENTS PER SERVING:
Calories: 505
Protein: 40 grams
Fat: 13 grams
Carbohydrate: 57 grams

1 cup	wild rice
2 Tbsp	butter
4	shallots, finely chopped
1 cup	dry white wine
1 cup	orange juice
2 tsp	grated orange rind
	Salt and pepper
	Clear honey
8	lemon sole fillets
2 Tbsp	all-purpose flour
	Oil
2	oranges, peeled and cut into segments, membranes removed
2 Tbsp	chopped fresh parsley

◆ In a large saucepan of boiling salted water, cook the rice for 40 to 45 minutes, or until tender.

◆ In a large saucepan, melt the butter. Add the shallots, and cook for 3 minutes.

◆ Add the wine, orange juice, and orange rind. Bring to a boil and continue boiling until reduced by half. Season with salt and pepper to taste. Add honey to taste. Cover and keep warm.

◆ Coat the fillets with the flour, and season well. In a frying pan, heat the oil. Add the fish in batches, and cook for 3 minutes on each side, or until fish is opaque. Keep warm.

◆ Drain the rice. Stir in the orange segments. Spoon the rice onto a warmed serving dish, and place the fish on top. Pour the sauce over the fish, and garnish with parsley.

Scallops WITH White Wine AND Tarragon Sauce

{ MAKES 4 SERVINGS }

Enjoy tender scallops in a creamy herb and wine sauce—without the cream! Serve with rice or pasta.

THIS RECIPE IS *FREE* OF THE FOLLOWING TRIGGERS

Caffeine ✓

Chocolate ✓

Citrus fruits ✓

Red wine ✓

Aged cheese ✓

MSG & nitrates ✓

Aspartame ✓

Nuts ✓

Onions & garlic

Yeast ✓

NUTRIENTS PER SERVING:
Calories: 215
Protein: 23 grams
Fat: 7 grams
Carbohydrate: 15 grams

1 lb	large sea scallops (about 16)
2 Tbsp	margarine, divided
½ cup	diced shallots
½ cup	diced carrots
2 Tbsp	minced sweet red pepper
1	clove garlic, minced
2 Tbsp	all-purpose flour
½ cup	dry white wine
1 cup	2% milk
2 Tbsp	chopped fresh parsley
1 Tbsp	chopped fresh tarragon
	Salt and pepper
2 Tbsp	chopped chives

♦ Rinse the scallops under cold water, and dry with paper towels.

♦ In a large skillet over medium heat, melt 1 tablespoon of the margarine. Cook the scallops for 1 minute per side. Remove, and set aside.

♦ Melt the remaining margarine. Add the shallots, carrots, and red pepper; sauté for 5 minutes. Stir in the garlic; sauté for 1 minute. Stir in the flour; cook for 1 minute. Pour in the wine, stirring constantly.

♦ Gradually add the milk, stirring constantly, until the sauce comes to a boil. Reduce the heat and simmer, stirring occasionally, for 3 minutes.

♦ Stir in the scallops, parsley, and tarragon. Cook for 30 seconds. Season to taste with salt and pepper. Pour into a serving dish, or spoon onto plates and garnish with the chives.

{ **VARIATION:** Substitute fresh dill for the tarragon. }

Grilled Shrimp WITH Two Marinades

{ MAKES 4 SERVINGS }

If you enjoy the delicate flavors of orange and sesame, then you'll love the orange-sesame marinade. If you're in the mood for something a little more assertive, the zestiness of balsamic vinegar might be just the thing.

THIS RECIPE IS *FREE* OF THE FOLLOWING TRIGGERS

Caffeine ✓

Chocolate ✓

Citrus fruits

Red wine ✓

Aged cheese ✓

MSG & nitrates

Aspartame ✓

Nuts ✓

Onions & garlic

Yeast ✓

NUTRIENTS PER SERVING:
Calories: 45
Protein: 7 grams
Fat: 1 gram
Carbohydrate: 2 grams

| 20 | medium or large shrimp, shelled and deveined, with tails intact |

ORANGE-SESAME MARINADE

3 Tbsp	orange juice concentrate
1 tsp	sesame oil
	Pepper

BALSAMIC VINEGAR AND GARLIC MARINADE

2 Tbsp	olive oil
1½ tsp	balsamic vinegar
½ tsp	Worcestershire sauce
1	clove garlic, minced
	Cayenne pepper

- In a glass bowl, mix the ingredients for the marinade of your choice.

- Add the shrimp, and toss to coat. Marinate for 1 hour at room temperature.

- Grill over medium heat, turning frequently, for about 5 minutes, or until the shrimp are bright pink. Do not over-cook.

Portuguese Seafood Risotto

{ MAKES 4 TO 6 SERVINGS }

A delectable combination of fresh shellfish and firm white fish, this creamy rice dish is best served with generous slices of fresh crusty bread.

THIS RECIPE IS *FREE* OF THE FOLLOWING TRIGGERS

Caffeine ✓

Chocolate ✓

Citrus fruits

Red wine ✓

Aged cheese ✓

MSG & nitrates ✓

Aspartame ✓

Nuts ✓

Onions & garlic

Yeast ✓

NUTRIENTS PER SERVING
(when serving 6):

Calories: 662

Protein: 41 grams

Fat: 38 grams

Carbohydrate: 39 grams

½ cup	olive oil
1	onion, finely chopped
3	cloves garlic, finely chopped
18	large mussels, scrubbed and bearded
12	medium shrimp, shelled and deveined
6	medium to large clams, scrubbed
¾ lb	salmon fillet
¾ lb	monkfish, cubed
2	squid, cleaned and cut into rings
1 ¼ cups	arborio rice
1 cup	white wine (optional)
2 cups	Fish Stock (see p. 119) or water
Pinch	saffron
	Salt and pepper
⅓ cup	butter
1 Tbsp	chopped coriander
1 Tbsp	lemon juice

♦ In a large, deep sauté pan or casserole, heat the olive oil over medium-high heat. Add the onion, garlic, and all of the shellfish and fish; cook for 2 to 3 minutes. Remove from the heat, and set aside all the shellfish and fish. Discard any clams and mussels that do not open.

♦ Add the rice to the mixture remaining in the pan. Stir for 2 minutes. Do not allow the rice to brown. Add the wine, if using, and allow it to evaporate over high heat.

♦ Reduce the heat to medium. Add the stock or water in small amounts, adding more as the liquid is absorbed. Add the saffron and salt and pepper to taste. Stir constantly until the rice has a creamy texture and is tender but firm, approximately 12 to 15 minutes. Add additional liquid, if necessary.

◆ Add the shellfish and fish to the risotto and cook for 3 minutes, or until heated through. Gently stir in the butter, coriander, and lemon juice. Adjust the seasoning, if necessary.

KITCHEN POINTER: Clams and mussels should be removed as soon as they unclench their shells, otherwise they will become tough. Some shells will open up sooner than others, and the mussels will open up before the clams. Clam and mussel shells that do not open should be discarded.

Shrimp AND Carrot Risotto

{ MAKES 4 SERVINGS }

Here's a risotto recipe that combines the earthiness of arborio rice with tender morsels of shrimp and cooked carrot for a dash of color.

NUTRIENTS PER SERVING:
Calories: 532
Protein: 14 grams
Fat: 16 grams
Carbohydrate: 83 grams

3	carrots, peeled and chopped
	Salt and pepper
2 Tbsp	olive oil
3	shallots, peeled and sliced
1½ cups	arborio rice
½ cup	carrot cooking liquid (reserved from step #2)
3 cups	Vegetable Stock (see p. 117)
1 cup	carrots, peeled and grated
3 Tbsp	unsalted butter
16	medium shrimp, peeled, deveined, and precooked
	Fresh Italian parsley, chopped

- In a large saucepan, cover the chopped carrots with water. Add a pinch of salt. Bring to a boil; reduce the heat, and simmer for about 20 minutes, or until tender.

- Strain the carrots, and reserve ½ cup of the cooking liquid for later. In a food processor, puree the cooked carrots until smooth. Place in a bowl, and set aside.

- In a large saucepan, heat the olive oil over medium-high heat. Add the shallots, and cook for about 3 minutes.

- Add the rice, and continue to cook for another 3 minutes. Add the carrot cooking liquid, and simmer, stirring occasionally, until the liquid has been absorbed.

- Add 1½ cups of the vegetable stock, stirring occasionally, until the liquid has been absorbed.

- Stir in the carrot puree, the grated carrot, and the remaining stock. Simmer, stirring, until the liquid is absorbed and the risotto has a creamy texture. Add the butter and shrimp; stir until the butter is incorporated and the shrimp are heated through. Serve on individual dinner plates or on a large serving platter. Garnish with the parsley.

Vegetables

AND Side Dishes

Stir-Fried Peppers AND Sprouts

{ MAKES 2 SERVINGS }

This simple and colorful side dish features bright red and green peppers fried with the tanginess of fresh ginger and bean sprouts.

THIS RECIPE IS *FREE* OF THE FOLLOWING TRIGGERS

Caffeine ✓

Chocolate ✓

Citrus fruits ✓

Red wine ✓

Aged cheese ✓

MSG & nitrates ✓

Aspartame ✓

Nuts ✓

Onions & garlic

Yeast ✓

NUTRIENTS PER SERVING:

Calories: 156

Protein: 4 grams

Fat: 12 grams

Carbohydrate: 8 grams

2 Tbsp	cooking oil
1 tsp	minced ginger root
½ tsp	salt
1	green pepper, cut in strips
1	red pepper, cut in strips
¾ lb	fresh bean sprouts
¼ cup	Chicken Stock (see p. 118)

◆ In a wok or skillet, heat the oil. Add the ginger, salt, and peppers. Stir-fry for 2 minutes. Add the bean sprouts, and stir-fry for 1 minute. Add the stock, cover, and cook for 2 to 3 minutes, or until the vegetables are tender.

Roasted Vegetable Medley

{ MAKES ABOUT 4 SERVINGS }

Roasted in their own juices, these vegetables are tender and very flavorful.

THIS RECIPE IS *FREE* OF THE FOLLOWING TRIGGERS

Caffeine ✓

Chocolate ✓

Citrus fruits ✓

Red wine ✓

Aged cheese ✓

MSG & nitrates ✓

Aspartame ✓

Nuts ✓

Onions & garlic

Yeast ✓

NUTRIENTS PER SERVING:
Calories: 218
Protein: 5 grams
Fat: 6 grams
Carbohydrate: 36 grams

6	small red potatoes (peeled if desired), quartered
4	large carrots (peeled if desired), cut into 3" lengths
2	small yellow onions, peeled and quartered
2 Tbsp	olive oil
2	small zucchini, cut into ½" slices
1 tsp	thyme
	Salt and pepper

◆ Preheat the oven to 425°F. In a bowl, combine the potatoes, carrots, and onions, and toss with 1½ tablespoon of the olive oil. In a separate bowl, toss the zucchini with the remaining oil. Place all the vegetables (except the zucchini) in a roasting pan. Sprinkle with the thyme and salt and pepper to taste. Roast for about 40 minutes. Add the zucchini, and gently turn the vegetables. Roast for another 15 to 20 minutes, or until the vegetables are tender.

{ **VARIATIONS:** Parsnips, turnips, fennel, chunks of celery root, and winter squash also make good vegetables for roasting. Garlic and herbs such as bay leaves can be added for additional flavor. }

Asparagus Spears WITH Apple, Egg, AND Poppy Seed Dressing

{ MAKES 4 SERVINGS }

This dish is best made in late spring or early summer, when asparagus is at its peak. A perfect accompaniment to grilled meats, it also works well as part of an antipasto plate. Make sure you have hard-boiled eggs on hand for this recipe.

THIS RECIPE IS *FREE* OF THE FOLLOWING TRIGGERS

Caffeine ✓

Chocolate ✓

Citrus fruits ✓

Red wine ✓

Aged cheese ✓

MSG & nitrates ✓

Aspartame ✓

Nuts ✓

Onions & garlic ✓

Yeast ✓

NUTRIENTS PER SERVING:
Calories: 131
Protein: 6 grams
Fat: 3 grams
Carbohydrate: 20 grams

24	spears fresh asparagus
2 or 3	hard-boiled eggs
1 cup	apple juice
½ cup	apple cider vinegar (approx.)
2 Tbsp	honey
1 Tbsp	poppy seeds

- Wash the asparagus; snap off the tough ends, and peel the remaining stems. In a large skillet of boiling water, blanch the asparagus for about 15 to 20 seconds, or until barely tender. Immediately immerse the asparagus in ice water to stop the cooking process. Set aside.

- Peel the eggs, and separate the yolks from the whites. Grate the yolks into a bowl. Add the apple juice, apple cider vinegar, honey, and poppy seeds. Whisk, using only as much cider vinegar as required to make a pourable sauce.

- Dice the egg whites. Reheat the asparagus in hot water; drain, and place six spears per person on individual salad plates. Pour the sauce over the asparagus, and decorate with the diced egg whites.

Charred Zucchini
with Herbs, Garlic, and Ricotta

{ MAKES 4 SERVINGS }

Salting and draining the zucchini prevents excess liquid from watering down this light and tasty side dish.

NUTRIENTS PER SERVING:

Calories: 89

Protein: 5 grams

Fat: 5 grams

Carbohydrate: 6 grams

2	medium green or yellow zucchini
	Salt
1 tsp	olive oil
2	stems fresh thyme
Pinch	dried oregano
1 Tbsp	fresh chopped basil and/or Italian parsley
2	cloves garlic, minced
½ cup	fresh ricotta cheese or goat cheese
1 tsp	dry bread crumbs
1 tsp	melted butter

♦ Cut the zucchini in half lengthwise. Sprinkle with salt, and let sit for about 20 minutes. Dry the zucchini with paper towels, and coat with the olive oil.

♦ Grill or broil the zucchini halves on high heat for about 3 minutes. Toss immediately with the herbs and garlic. Let cool slightly; slice. In an ovenproof dish, toss with the ricotta. Top with the bread crumbs and butter. Place under a broiler to melt the cheese. Serve immediately.

{ **KITCHEN POINTER:** Be sure not to overcook the zucchini, or the entire dish will become soggy. }

Roasted New Potatoes WITH Herbs

In this side dish, new red potatoes are perfectly offset by a delicate combination of garlic, rosemary, and thyme. Serve with roasted chicken, turkey, or pork.

THIS RECIPE IS *FREE* OF THE FOLLOWING TRIGGERS

Caffeine ✓

Chocolate ✓

Citrus fruits ✓

Red wine ✓

Aged cheese ✓

MSG & nitrates ✓

Aspartame ✓

Nuts ✓

Onions & garlic

Yeast ✓

NUTRIENTS PER SERVING:
Calories: 248
Protein: 4 grams
Fat: 12 grams
Carbohydrate: 31 grams

3 lbs	new red potatoes, quartered
6 Tbsp	olive oil or canola oil
3	cloves garlic, minced
1 Tbsp	each dried rosemary and thyme
1 tsp	dried oregano
	Salt and pepper

- In a large bowl, combine the potatoes, oil, and garlic; toss to coat. Add the herbs, and toss again. Season with salt and pepper to taste. Divide the potatoes between 2 large, heavy baking sheets. Bake at 500°F for about 30 minutes, or until brown and crisp, stirring occasionally.

Mushrooms AND Rice

{ MAKES 6 SERVINGS }

The earthy texture of rice is a perfect match with fresh mushrooms. Serve this quick-cooking side dish with your favorite grilled meats.

THIS RECIPE IS *FREE* OF THE FOLLOWING TRIGGERS

Caffeine ✓

Chocolate ✓

Citrus fruits ✓

Red wine ✓

Aged cheese ✓

MSG & nitrates ✓

Aspartame ✓

Nuts ✓

Onions & garlic ✓

Yeast ✓

NUTRIENTS PER SERVING:
Calories: 171
Protein: 3 grams
Fat: 7 grams
Carbohydrate: 24 grams

¼ cup	butter
½ cup	finely chopped onion
¼ cup	finely chopped celery
3 cups	sliced mushrooms
½ tsp	each dried thyme and sage
	Cooked rice (enough for 6 servings)
	Fresh parsley, chopped
	Salt and pepper

◆ In a large skillet, melt the butter over medium heat. Cook the onion and celery until soft. Add the mushrooms, thyme, and sage. Cook, stirring, for 3 to 4 minutes. Add the mixture to the cooked rice; stir in the parsley. Salt and pepper to taste.

Steamed Basmati Rice
WITH Crisp Potatoes, Sumac, AND Cumin

{ MAKES 6 TO 8 SERVINGS }

Fragrant basmati tops a layer of crispy sweet potatoes in this Middle Eastern–inspired side dish.

THIS RECIPE IS *FREE* OF THE FOLLOWING TRIGGERS

Caffeine ✓

Chocolate ✓

Citrus fruits ✓

Red wine ✓

Aged cheese ✓

MSG & nitrates ✓

Aspartame ✓

Nuts ✓

Onions & garlic ✓

Yeast ✓

NUTRIENTS PER SERVING
(when serving 8):

Calories: 341
Protein: 5 grams
Fat: 9 grams
Carbohydrate: 60 grams

1 lb	basmati rice
⅓ cup	olive oil
3	sweet potatoes, peeled and sliced ¼" thick
1	lemon zest, cut in thin strips
1 Tbsp	each ground cumin and sumac
	Salt and pepper

• In a large saucepan of boiling water, cook the rice for about 10 minutes, or until about half cooked. Strain off the water, and set aside.

• Place 2 tablespoons of the olive oil in a stainless steel pot with a lid. Arrange the sweet potato slices side by side to cover the entire bottom of the pot. Begin scooping rice into the center of the pot to form a dome shape. Once all the rice is in, lightly pat it down, maintaining the shape within ¼" of the edges. Put breather holes in the rice, penetrating down to the bottom. Lightly drizzle the rice with the remaining olive oil, and season with lemon zest, cumin, sumac, and salt and pepper to taste.

• Place a damp dish towel over the pot, put the lid on, and place the pot on the stove. Cook over medium-high heat for about 7 minutes, or until the potatoes are crispy.

• Serve immediately.

Wild Cherry Tabbouleh

{ MAKES 4 TO 6 SERVINGS }

The nuttiness of bulgur is perfectly offset by the sweetness of cherries in this dish. Serve with your favorite grilled meats or as a main course salad with some bread. This salad makes an excellent addition to any picnic basket, because it should be served at room temperature.

THIS RECIPE IS *FREE* OF THE FOLLOWING TRIGGERS

Caffeine ✓

Chocolate ✓

Citrus fruits ✓

Red wine ✓

Aged cheese ✓

MSG & nitrates ✓

Aspartame ✓

Nuts ✓

Onions & garlic ✓

Yeast ✓

NUTRIENTS PER SERVING
(when serving 6):

Calories: 109
Protein: 3 grams
Fat: 1 gram
Carbohydrate: 22 grams

MAKE AHEAD: The tabbouleh can be prepared earlier in the day or a day in advance. Store in the refrigerator, and bring to room temperature before serving.

1 cup	bulgur
2 cups	boiling water or Chicken Stock (see p. 118)
2 cups	fresh cherries, pitted and split
2 Tbsp	each chopped fresh mint and parsley
	Salt and pepper
	Sunflower oil

- In a medium bowl, gradually add the boiling water or stock to the bulgur until it has absorbed enough liquid to allow it to swell and become tender, but not soggy.

- Add the cherries, mint, parsley, and salt and pepper to taste. Mix thoroughly. Let stand for approximately 30 minutes in a cool place.

- Add more water or stock as needed, as well as sunflower oil, if desired.

- Kitchen Pointer: Cherry pitters are available at kitchen supply stores. This gadget makes pitting cherries easier than having to cut them in half and then prying out the pit.

Bulgur and Green Bean Salad
WITH Herbed Vinaigrette

{ MAKES 6 TO 8 SERVINGS }

Bulgur is parboiled cracked wheat that is easy to prepare. It has a nutty flavor and a pleasant, chewy texture.

THIS RECIPE IS *FREE* OF THE FOLLOWING TRIGGERS

Caffeine ✓

Chocolate ✓

Citrus fruits ✓

Red wine ✓

Aged cheese ✓

MSG & nitrates ✓

Aspartame ✓

Nuts ✓

Onions & garlic

Yeast ✓

NUTRIENTS PER SERVING
(when serving 8):

Calories: 336
Protein: 12 grams
Fat: 16 grams
Carbohydrate: 36 grams

2 cups	bulgur
2 cups	boiling water
¾ lb	green beans
⅓ cup	balsamic vinegar (or cider vinegar and 1 tsp brown sugar)
3	cloves garlic, minced
1 tsp	each chopped fresh thyme, oregano, and rosemary
1 cup	olive oil or canola oil
	Salt and pepper
3	medium tomatoes, chopped
1 cup	chopped, pitted kalamata olives
4 cups	mixed greens
½ lb	soft mild goat cheese, crumbled

• In a large bowl, combine the bulgur and water. Set aside.

• In a saucepan, cook the green beans in boiling salted water for about 4 minutes, or until tender but crisp. Drain well. Pat dry. Add to the bulgur.

• In a medium bowl, combine the vinegar, garlic, and herbs. Gradually whisk in the oil. Season to taste with salt and pepper.

• Add the tomatoes and olives to the bulgur. Mix in enough vinaigrette to coat completely. Season with salt and pepper to taste.

• Mound the mixed greens on a platter. Top with the bulgur, and add the goat cheese as garnish.

{ **KITCHEN POINTER:** Chicken can be added to this dish to make a complete meal. }

Grilled Polenta
WITH Tomato Sauce

{ MAKES 4 TO 6 SERVINGS }

In this recipe, the polenta is allowed to harden, then it's sliced, grilled, and served with tomato sauce to make a zesty side dish.

THIS RECIPE IS *FREE* OF THE FOLLOWING TRIGGERS

Caffeine ✓

Chocolate ✓

Citrus fruits ✓

Red wine ✓

Aged cheese ✓

MSG & nitrates ✓

Aspartame ✓

Nuts ✓

Onions & garlic

Yeast ✓

NUTRIENTS PER SERVING
(when serving 6):

Calories: 353

Protein: 12 grams

Fat: 9 grams

Carbohydrate: 56 grams

MAKE AHEAD: The polenta can be prepared and refrigerated up to a day in advance. Grill prior to serving.

2 Tbsp	vegetable oil or butter
2	shallots, diced
½ cup	fresh corn (whole kernels)
1	red pepper, diced
1 tsp	finely chopped garlic
4 cups	milk
4 cups	Chicken Stock (see p. 118)
2 cups	fine cornmeal
1 Tbsp	each chopped fresh mixed herbs (rosemary, thyme, etc.)
½	lemon, juiced
	Salt and pepper
¾ cup	tomato sauce
6 sprigs	fresh rosemary or thyme

◆ In a large saucepan, heat the oil. Cook the shallots until tender. Add the corn, red pepper, and garlic; cook until tender.

◆ Add the milk and stock; bring to a boil over medium heat. Slowly whisk in the cornmeal. Add the herbs, lemon juice, and salt and pepper to taste. Cook for an additional 5 to 10 minutes, or until creamy and thick.

◆ Pour the polenta into a 9″ square cake pan lined with plastic wrap. Gently tap the pan to ensure that the polenta gets into all corners. Let cool. Cover, and refrigerate for 2 hours (or overnight).

◆ To serve, unmold the polenta and remove the plastic wrap. Slice into ¼″ or ½″ pieces, and cut on the diagonal to form two triangles. On a preheated grill, grill the polenta until heated through, turning once.

◆ Meanwhile, in a saucepan over medium-low heat, heat the tomato sauce. Spoon some sauce onto individual plates. Arrange two triangles per person on top. Garnish with a sprig of rosemary or thyme.

{ **KITCHEN POINTER:** If fresh corn is unavailable, frozen or canned whole kernels can be substituted. }

Basic Stocks

AND Sauces

Vegetable Stock

{ MAKES ABOUT 12 CUPS }

Here's a flavorful meatless stock that will keep in the refrigerator for one week. Or it can be frozen for later use.

THIS RECIPE IS *FREE* OF THE FOLLOWING TRIGGERS

Caffeine ✓

Chocolate ✓

Citrus fruits ✓

Red wine ✓

Aged cheese ✓

MSG & nitrates ✓

Aspartame ✓

Nuts ✓

Onions & garlic

Yeast ✓

NUTRIENTS:
Contains less than 10 calories per 1 cup and trace amounts of protein, fat, and carbohydrates.

1 Tbsp	olive oil
3 cups	sliced carrots
3 cups	sliced onions
2 cups	chopped savoy cabbage
2 cups	sliced leeks
1½ cups	sliced celery
1 cup	peeled and sliced parsnips
½ cup	parsley sprigs
3	cloves garlic
2	fresh thyme sprigs
2 Tbsp	chopped fresh basil
1	bay leaf
1 tsp	whole black peppercorns
2 tsp	kosher sea salt
1	medium potato, sliced
2	medium tomatoes, chopped
12 cups	water

◆ In a stockpot over medium-high heat, heat the olive oil. Add the remaining ingredients except the potato, tomatoes, and water. Cook, stirring occasionally, for about 6 to 8 minutes, or until the vegetables soften.

◆ Add the potato, tomatoes, and water. Bring to a boil; lower the heat, and simmer, covered, for 40 minutes. Strain the stock through a colander over a bowl, pressing down on the vegetables to extract as much stock as possible.

◆ Refrigerate to cool. Once the stock is cold, it should be tightly covered.

Chicken OR Beef Stock

{ MAKES 12 TO 16 CUPS }

Canned soups and powdered stock mixes often contain MSG or other preservatives that can be triggers. Fortunately, a flavorful chicken or beef stock is not difficult to make. If onions and garlic are triggers for you, they can be omitted from the recipe.

THIS RECIPE IS *FREE* OF THE FOLLOWING TRIGGERS

Caffeine ✓

Chocolate ✓

Citrus fruits ✓

Red wine ✓

Aged cheese ✓

MSG & nitrates ✓

Aspartame ✓

Nuts ✓

Onions & garlic

Yeast ✓

NUTRIENTS:
Contains less than 10 calories per 1 cup and trace amounts of protein, fat, and carbohydrates.

	Beef or chicken bones (enough to fill an 8-quart pot; brown beef bones first for richer broth)
2 cups	chopped celery
2	medium carrots, chopped
2	medium onions, chopped
½ tsp	each oregano and thyme
2 tsp	chopped fresh parsley
2	bay leaves
2	cloves garlic
1 Tbsp	salt
8	peppercorns
4	whole cloves

• Place the bones in a stockpot over medium-high heat. Add all the remaining ingredients, and cover with water. (If omitting onions and garlic, add extra bay leaf and another carrot or parsnip.) Bring to a boil; lower the heat, and simmer, covered, for 4 to 6 hours. Strain in a colander over a large bowl. Discard the bones and vegetables. Refrigerate overnight; remove the fat.

{ KITCHEN POINTER: This stock can be stored in batches in the freezer and used as the base for many homemade soups. }

Fish Stock

{ MAKES ABOUT 12 CUPS }

This versatile stock can be refrigerated for up to five days or frozen for up to six months.

THIS RECIPE IS *FREE* OF THE FOLLOWING TRIGGERS

Caffeine ✓

Chocolate ✓

Citrus fruits

Red wine ✓

Aged cheese ✓

MSG & nitrates ✓

Aspartame ✓

Nuts ✓

Onions & garlic

Yeast ✓

NUTRIENTS:
Contains less than 10 calories per 1 cup and trace amounts of protein, fat, and carbohydrates.

12 cups	water
1 cup	dry white wine
4 lbs	fish trimmings, washed
2	celery sticks, sliced
1	onion, sliced
2 Tbsp	lemon juice
6	peppercorns
4 sprigs	fresh parsley
2 sprigs	fresh thyme or ½ tsp dried

- In a stockpot, bring the water and wine to a boil over high heat. Add the fish trimmings, celery, and onion.

- Add the remaining ingredients. When the water returns to a boil, reduce the heat so that the stock is barely simmering; simmer for 2½ to 3 hours.

- Strain the stock, extracting as much liquid as possible. Discard the solids, and let the stock reach room temperature before refrigerating or freezing.

Hollandaise Sauce

{ MAKES ABOUT 2 CUPS }

Serve this sauce over Poached Salmon (see p. 89), eggs Benedict, or asparagus.

THIS RECIPE IS *FREE* OF THE FOLLOWING TRIGGERS

Caffeine ✓

Chocolate ✓

Citrus fruits

Red wine ✓

Aged cheese ✓

MSG & nitrates ✓

Aspartame ✓

Nuts ✓

Onions & garlic ✓

Yeast ✓

NUTRIENTS PER SERVING
(2 Tbsp):

Calories: 103

Protein: 1 gram

Fat: 11 grams

Carbohydrate: trace

6	egg yolks
2 Tbsp	lemon juice
½ lb	butter, melted
¼ cup	hot water
Pinch	cayenne pepper
	Salt

+ In the top of a double boiler or in a metal bowl placed over a saucepan of hot (but not simmering) water, beat the egg yolks with a wire whisk until smooth.

+ Add the lemon juice, and gradually whisk in the melted butter, pouring in a thin stream.

+ Slowly stir in the hot water, cayenne pepper, and salt to taste. Continue to mix for about 1 minute, or until the sauce is thickened.

+ Serve immediately.

Homemade Soy Sauce

Most commercially made soy sauces contain MSG, a common trigger for migraine. If you cannot find naturally brewed soy sauce, you might want to consider this recipe for concentrated beef broth. This sauce can be used as a substitute for soy sauce.

THIS RECIPE IS *FREE* OF THE FOLLOWING TRIGGERS

Caffeine ✓

Chocolate ✓

Citrus fruits ✓

Red wine ✓

Aged cheese ✓

MSG & nitrates ✓

Aspartame ✓

Nuts ✓

Onions & garlic ✓

Yeast ✓

NUTRIENTS PER SERVING:
One tablespoon contains less than 10 calories and very small amounts of protein and carbohydrate.

¾ cup	beef drippings
¼ cup	water
	Sea salt optional

- Next time you make roast beef, instead of making gravy, save the drippings. After the drippings are cool, make sure to skim off the fat.

- In a bowl, mix the drippings with the water. Add sea salt, if desired.

- Store this sauce in an airtight container in the freezer for up to three months.

Quick Breads

Never-Fail Biscuits

{ MAKES ABOUT 15 BISCUITS }
(USING A 2″ ROUND CUTTER)

These fluffy white biscuits are an excellent accompaniment to any meal. They can also be served simply with butter and jam.

THIS RECIPE IS *FREE* OF THE FOLLOWING TRIGGERS

Caffeine ✓

Chocolate ✓

Citrus fruits ✓

Red wine ✓

Aged cheese ✓

MSG & nitrates ✓

Aspartame ✓

Nuts ✓

Onions & garlic ✓

Yeast ✓

NUTRIENTS PER SERVING:
Calories: 131
Protein: 3 grams
Fat: 7 grams
Carbohydrate: 14 grams

2 cups	all-purpose flour
4 tsp	baking powder
1 tsp	granulated sugar
½ tsp	salt
½ cup	margarine
⅔ cup	milk
1	egg

• In a large bowl, blend together the flour, baking powder, sugar, and salt. Finely cut in the margarine. Add the milk and egg; mix well. Place the dough on a lightly floured surface, and roll or pat to the desired thickness. Cut with a floured round biscuit cutter.

• Tranfer the rounds to a lightly greased baking sheet. Bake at 450°F for 10 to 12 minutes, or until lightly browned.

Healthy Biscuits

{ MAKES ABOUT 12 BISCUITS }

Spelt is a type of wheat. The combination of spelt and oat flours produces a surprisingly light biscuit with a rich, nutty flavor. This recipe can be doubled with good results.

THIS RECIPE IS *FREE* OF THE FOLLOWING TRIGGERS

Caffeine ✓

Chocolate ✓

Citrus fruits ✓

Red wine ✓

Aged cheese ✓

MSG & nitrates ✓

Aspartame ✓

Nuts ✓

Onions & garlic ✓

Yeast ✓

NUTRIENTS PER SERVING:
Calories: 181
Protein: 4 grams
Fat: 9 grams
Carbohydrate: 21 grams

1¼ cups	spelt flour
1¼ cups	oat flour
2 tsp	baking powder
¼ tsp	baking soda
¼ tsp	sea salt
½ cup	butter
¾ cup	buttermilk

♦ In a large bowl, combine the flours, baking powder, baking soda, and salt; cut in the butter until the mixture resembles coarse crumbs (using your hands usually works best for this). Stir in the buttermilk to form a soft dough.

♦ Turn it out onto a lightly floured surface, and knead gently. Roll out to about ½" thickness. and cut into 2½" rounds with a biscuit cutter. In a pinch, a drinking glass can even be used for this purpose. Transfer to a lightly greased baking sheet, and bake at 375°F for about 10 minutes, or until just golden on top. (Watch carefully; every oven is different.)

{ **VARIATIONS:** This biscuit can be baked as a sweet bread (scone) by adding 1 teaspoon sugar and ¼ cup raisins or chopped candied ginger. For savory biscuits, add chopped fresh herbs or dry herbs. }

Irish Scones

Made with rolled oats and raisins, these are a nutritious and tasty alternative to ordinary scones.

THIS RECIPE IS *FREE* OF THE FOLLOWING TRIGGERS

Caffeine ✓

Chocolate ✓

Citrus fruits ✓

Red wine ✓

Aged cheese ✓

MSG & nitrates ✓

Aspartame ✓

Nuts ✓

Onions & garlic ✓

Yeast ✓

NUTRIENTS PER SERVING:
Calories: 194
Protein: 4 grams
Fat: 6 grams
Carbohydrate: 31 grams

2½ cups	all-purpose flour
¼ cup	rolled oats
2 Tbsp	granulated sugar
2 tsp	baking powder
2 tsp	baking soda
½ tsp	salt
⅓ cup	shortening or butter
1¼ cups	milk
½ cup	raisins

- Mix together the flour, oats, sugar, baking powder, baking soda, and salt. With a pastry blender or two knives, cut in the shortening or butter. Add the milk, and stir in the raisins.

- Turn the dough out onto a lightly floured surface. Pat or roll it out to ¾" thickness. Cut into rounds using a 2" cutter. Bake at 400°F for 10 to 15 minutes, or until golden brown.

> **KITCHEN POINTER:** The secret to light and fluffy biscuits or scones is to work the dough as little as possible. Pastry or baking soda dough toughens the more you work it, because the gluten in the flour is activated.

Buttermilk Scones

{ MAKES ABOUT 12 SCONES }

A healthy alternative to sweet scones, these can also be served as a savory appetizer with your favorite cheese.

THIS RECIPE IS *FREE* OF THE FOLLOWING TRIGGERS

Caffeine ✓

Chocolate ✓

Citrus fruits ✓

Red wine ✓

Aged cheese ✓

MSG & nitrates ✓

Aspartame ✓

Nuts ✓

Onions & garlic ✓

Yeast ✓

NUTRIENTS PER SERVING:
Calories: 129
Protein: 4 grams
Fat: 1 gram
Carbohydrate: 26 grams

3 cups	all-purpose flour
1 Tbsp	baking powder
1½ tsp	salt
1–2 cups	buttermilk

♦ In a large bowl, sift together the flour, baking powder, and salt. Gradually add the buttermilk until the dough is stiff.

♦ Turn it out onto a lightly floured board, and roll out to about ¾″ thickness. Cut with a large round cookie cutter. Bake at 350°F on an ungreased griddle or a greased baking sheet for about 25 minutes, or until golden brown.

Corn Bread

{ MAKES ABOUT 12 TO 16 SERVINGS }

Sure to bring back memories of home, this corn bread is wonderful accompanied by a bowl of steaming chili.

THIS RECIPE IS *FREE* OF THE FOLLOWING TRIGGERS

Caffeine ✓

Chocolate ✓

Citrus fruits ✓

Red wine ✓

Aged cheese ✓

MSG & nitrates ✓

Aspartame ✓

Nuts ✓

Onions & garlic ✓

Yeast ✓

NUTRIENTS PER SERVING:
Calories: 260
Protein: 3 grams
Fat: 16 grams
Carbohydrate: 26 grams

2 cups	biscuit mix
1 cup	cornmeal
¾ cup	granulated sugar
½ tsp	baking soda
½ tsp	salt
1 cup	light cream
1 cup	margarine
2	eggs, lightly beaten

• In a large bowl, mix the biscuit mix, cornmeal, sugar, baking soda, and salt. In a saucepan, scald the cream with the margarine; add to the dry ingredients. Mix in the eggs.

• Pour the batter into a greased and floured 13″ × 9″ baking dish or pan, spreading evenly. Bake at 350°F for 30 minutes, or until lightly browned and firm to the touch. Let stand for several minutes before cutting.

Zucchini Bread

{ MAKES 2 LOAVES }

Rich, moist, fragrant, and delicious, zucchini bread is more of a treat than a bread. It's perfect for breakfast, as a snack, or for dessert.

THIS RECIPE IS *FREE* OF THE FOLLOWING TRIGGERS

Caffeine ✓

Chocolate ✓

Citrus fruits ✓

Red wine ✓

Aged cheese ✓

MSG & nitrates ✓

Aspartame ✓

Nuts ✓

Onions & garlic ✓

Yeast ✓

NUTRIENTS PER SERVING
(1 slice):

Calories: 135
Protein: 2 grams
Fat: 7 grams
Carbohydrate: 16 grams

3	eggs
2½ cups	grated zucchini
1 cup	butter, melted
1 cup	granulated sugar
3 cups	all-purpose flour
2 tsp	ground nutmeg
1 tsp	baking soda
1 tsp	cinnamon
1 tsp	salt
¼ tsp	baking powder

◆ In a large bowl, beat the eggs well. Blend in the zucchini, butter, and sugar.

◆ In a separate bowl, sift the flour, nutmeg, baking soda, cinnamon, salt, and baking powder. Stir into the zucchini mixture.

◆ Pour the batter into 2 greased loaf pans. Bake at 325°F for 1 hour, or until a tester inserted in the center comes out clean. Let cool in the pan for 10 minutes, then turn out onto a rack to cool completely.

VARIATION: Stir ½ cup raisins into the batter before pouring it into the pans.

Big Loonie Pancakes

Kids love these cakes served with sweetened strawberries or butter and maple syrup.

THIS RECIPE IS *FREE* OF THE FOLLOWING TRIGGERS

Caffeine ✓

Chocolate ✓

Citrus fruits ✓

Red wine ✓

Aged cheese ✓

MSG & nitrates ✓

Aspartame ✓

Nuts ✓

Onions & garlic ✓

Yeast ✓

NUTRIENTS PER SERVING:
Calories: 66
Protein: 3 grams
Fat: 2 grams
Carbohydrate: 9 grams

2	eggs, separated
¾–1 cup	milk
1 Tbsp	oil
1 cup	all-purpose flour

- In a large bowl, beat the egg whites until stiff. In a blender, blend the egg yolks. Add the milk to the yolks, and blend. Blend in the oil. Add the flour, and mix. Fold this mixture into the beaten egg whites.

- Heat a nonstick griddle to 400°F, or heat a nonstick skillet or griddle over medium heat. Using less than ¼ cup batter for each pancake, pour it onto the hot griddle. When the underside is brown and bubbles break on the top side, turn the pancake over and bake until the second side is golden.

Apple Pancakes

{ MAKES ABOUT 12 PANCAKES }

These tasty pancakes are ideal for a special-day breakfast.

NUTRIENTS PER SERVING:
Calories: 97
Protein: 3 grams
Fat: 1 gram
Carbohydrate: 19 grams

1½ cups	all-purpose flour
1 Tbsp	granulated sugar
1 Tbsp	baking powder
½ tsp	salt
1	egg, beaten
1½ cups	milk
2	small apples, finely chopped
1 tsp	cinnamon

◆ Mix together the flour, sugar, baking powder, and salt.

◆ In a separate bowl, mix the egg and milk; add to the dry mixture. Add the chopped apples and cinnamon, stirring only until the batter is moistened.

◆ Heat a nonstick skillet or griddle over medium heat. Pour the batter onto the griddle, using about ¼ cup for each pancake. When the underside is brown and bubbles break on the top side, turn the pancake over and continue cooking until the second side is golden brown. Serve with Apple Syrup (recipe follows).

APPLE SYRUP

1½ cups	chopped, peeled apple
¾ cup plus	apple juice (divided) 2 tsp
½ cup	maple syrup
2 tsp	cornstarch

◆ In a saucepan, combine the apples, ¾ cup apple juice, and maple syrup. Bring to a boil over medium heat, stirring occasionally. Reduce the heat, cover, and simmer for 10 minutes, or until the apples are tender.

◆ In a small bowl, combine the cornstarch and 2 teaspoons apple juice. Add to the hot mixture; cook, stirring, until slightly thickened. Serve warm over Apple Pancakes.

Desserts AND Baked Goods

Apple Cobbler

{ MAKES 2 TO 4 SERVINGS }

This delectable cobbler is made with rolled oats and is quick and easy to prepare. Serve it plain or with whipped cream or vanilla ice cream.

THIS RECIPE IS *FREE* OF THE FOLLOWING TRIGGERS

Caffeine ✓

Chocolate ✓

Citrus fruits ✓

Red wine ✓

Aged cheese ✓

MSG & nitrates ✓

Aspartame ✓

Nuts ✓

Onions & garlic ✓

Yeast ✓

Nutrients per serving
(when serving 4):
Calories: 706
Protein: 6 grams
Fat: 26 grams
Carbohydrate: 112 grams

MAKE AHEAD: The cobbler can be prepared several hours prior to serving and kept at room temperature.

3	Empire apples, peeled and cored
½ cup	apple juice
¼ cup	granulated sugar
1 Tbsp	cinnamon
1 tsp	nutmeg
1 cup	uncooked rolled oats
1 cup	brown sugar
½ cup	all-purpose flour
½ cup	unsalted butter

+ Cut the apples into ¼″ slices.

+ In a small saucepan, combine the apples, apple juice, granulated sugar, cinnamon, and nutmeg. Cook over medium heat for approximately 10 minutes, stirring occasionally, or until the mixture becomes syrupy.

+ In a bowl, mix the rolled oats, brown sugar, flour, and butter until thoroughly combined and the mixture resembles pea-sized shapes.

+ Pour the apple mixture into a 4″ deep baking dish (small loaf pan), and top evenly with the oat mixture. Bake at 400°F for approximately 4 to 5 minutes, or until the topping is browned and the fruit is bubbly.

Roasted Pears with Mint Anglaise

{ MAKES 4 SERVINGS }

Serve this elegant dessert garnished with fresh mint or with a scoop of your favorite ice cream.

THIS RECIPE IS *FREE* OF THE FOLLOWING TRIGGERS

Caffeine ✓

Chocolate ✓

Citrus fruits ✓

Red wine ✓

Aged cheese ✓

MSG & nitrates ✓

Aspartame ✓

Nuts ✓

Onions & garlic ✓

Yeast ✓

NUTRIENTS PER SERVING
(1 pear with ¼ cup sauce):
Calories: 225
Protein: 4 grams
Fat: 5 grams
Carbohydrate: 41 grams

MAKE AHEAD: The Mint Anglaise may be made up to 2 days in advance and stored in the refrigerator.

1 cup	granulated sugar
1 cup	water
4	Bartlett or Bosc pears, firm but ripe

SAUCE

8	egg yolks
1 cup	granulated sugar
2 tsp	cornstarch (optional)
4 cups	2% milk
1	bunch fresh mint, chopped + additional for garnish

- In a heavy saucepan, combine the sugar and water. Bring to a boil and let boil for several minutes only. Remove from the heat, and let cool. This makes a simple syrup.

- Peel and core the pears. Wrap the stems with aluminum foil. Cut the pears in a curvilinear pattern so that they will fan out on a plate. Dip the pears in the syrup.

- Arrange the pears on a greased baking sheet, and cook at 400°F for about 30 minutes, or until caramel in color.

To make the sauce:

- In a stainless steel bowl, whisk together the egg yolks and sugar. Beat in the cornstarch, if using. Set aside.

- In a saucepan, combine the milk and mint. Heat over medium heat, stirring occasionally. Bring the milk up to the boiling point, stirring often, but do not boil. Strain the milk. Gradually, in a thin stream, add the milk to the egg-sugar mixture while constantly whisking.

- In the top of a double boiler over simmering water or in a bowl over a saucepan filled with simmering water, cook the sauce, stirring constantly, until it coats the back of a spoon. Remove from the heat, and let cool.

- To serve, place some Mint Anglaise on dessert plates. Fan out a warm caramelized pear on each plate. Garnish with fresh mint.

Poached Fruit in Light Syrup
with Vanilla Ice Cream and Roasted Almonds

{ MAKES 4 SERVINGS }

This elegant and tasty dessert is sure to impress your guests. Vary the fruit to suit the season.

THIS RECIPE IS *FREE* OF THE FOLLOWING TRIGGERS

Caffeine ✓

Chocolate ✓

Citrus fruits ✓

Red wine ✓

Aged cheese ✓

MSG & nitrates ✓

Aspartame ✓

Nuts

Onions & garlic ✓

Yeast ✓

NUTRIENTS PER SERVING:
Calories: 380
Protein: 4 grams
Fat: 16 grams
Carbohydrate: 55 grams

2 cups	granulated sugar
4 cups	water
1	pear, cut into wedges
1	peach, cut into wedges
1 cup	fresh strawberries, hulled
8	scoops vanilla ice cream
¼ cup	slivered toasted almonds

◆ In a medium saucepan, combine the sugar and water to make a syrup. Bring to a boil and boil gently, stirring occasionally, for 5 minutes.

◆ Add the pear wedges to the syrup for 1 minute, then remove them. Add the peach wedges for 10 seconds; remove them. Add the strawberries for 10 seconds; remove them.

◆ Continue to boil the syrup until it reaches a slightly thick consistency.

◆ Meanwhile, in 4 champagne flutes, alternate layers of fruit and ice cream. Top with a sprinkling of almonds. Using a tablespoon, drizzle some of the syrup over the almonds. Serve immediately.

Allspice Roasted Bananas

{ MAKES 6 TO 8 SERVINGS }

A simple but tasty dessert; perfect with vanilla ice cream.

NUTRIENTS PER SERVING
(when serving 8):

Calories: 441

Protein: 1 gram

Fat: 13 grams

Carbohydrate: 80 grams

8	small to medium bananas
2 cups	firmly packed brown sugar
½ cup	unsalted butter, melted
5	whole allspice

◆ In a baking dish, top the whole peeled bananas with the brown sugar. Drizzle the melted butter evenly over the bananas and sugar. Scatter the allspice over the top.

◆ Bake at 425°F for about 10 minutes, or until the sugar melts, bubbles, and caramelizes, leaving the bananas soft.

◆ Serve over vanilla ice cream or yogurt.

{ **KITCHEN POINTER:** Watch the oven carefully, because bananas can burn quickly if left in too long. }

Blueberry Maple Pie
WITH Warmed Maple Syrup

{ MAKES 8 SERVINGS }

Maple syrup adds a delectable touch to this blueberry pie. It's perfect with vanilla ice cream.

THIS RECIPE IS *FREE* OF THE FOLLOWING TRIGGERS

Caffeine ✓

Chocolate ✓

Citrus fruits ✓

Red wine ✓

Aged cheese ✓

MSG & nitrates ✓

Aspartame ✓

Nuts ✓

Onions & garlic ✓

Yeast ✓

NUTRIENTS PER SERVING:
Calories: 480
Protein: 4 grams
Fat: 28 grams
Carbohydrate: 53 grams

MAKE AHEAD: Prepare the crust a day in advance. The pie can be baked earlier in the day and then warmed prior to serving.

CRUST

Pinch	salt
½ cup	cold water
1 Tbsp	maple syrup
1 cup	cold shortening
1½ cups	all-purpose flour
1	egg

FILLING

5 cups	fresh or frozen blueberries
½ cup	granulated sugar
¼ cup	maple syrup
2 Tbsp	cornstarch
¼ tsp	cinnamon

To make the crust:

• In a small bowl, dissolve the salt in the water. Add the maple syrup, and combine.

• In a large mixing bowl or food processor, work the shortening into the flour until the mixture resembles coarse meal with some larger pieces.

• Make a well in the center of the mixture. Gradually add the water mixture, using only as much as required to form dough. Without overhandling, knead the dough lightly and form it into a ball. Wrap in plastic wrap, and refrigerate for 30 minutes or overnight.

To make the filling:

- Cut the dough in 2 pieces. On a lightly floured surface, roll out 1 piece of dough into a round to fit a 9″ pie plate with a slight overhang. Roll out the second piece for the top crust.

- Line the bottom of a pie plate with dough, and gently press it into place. Trim the excess dough to the edge of the plate.

- Combine the blueberries, sugar, maple syrup, cornstarch, and cinnamon. Spread over the bottom crust.

- Cover with the top crust. Trim the sealing edges with egg wash (1 egg mixed with ½ eggshell of water).

- Make several slits in the dough to allow steam to vent. Brush the top with egg wash.

- Bake at 375°F until the juices bubble and the crust is golden.

- Serve warm or at room temperature with vanilla ice cream topped with warmed maple syrup.

Peach Tart

Artfully arranged atop a spongy cake and baked in the oven, peaches make an impressive dessert for entertaining. Try serving this with a dollop of whipped cream.

THIS RECIPE IS *FREE* OF THE FOLLOWING TRIGGERS

Caffeine ✓

Chocolate ✓

Citrus fruits

Red wine ✓

Aged cheese ✓

MSG & nitrates ✓

Aspartame ✓

Nuts ✓

Onions & garlic ✓

Yeast ✓

NUTRIENTS PER SERVING
(when serving 10):

Calories: 243
Protein: 3 grams
Fat: 11 grams
Carbohydrate: 33 grams

½ cup	butter
¾ cup	granulated sugar or brown sugar
1 cup	all-purpose flour or whole wheat flour
1 tsp	baking powder
Pinch	salt
2	eggs
4	peaches, sliced
¼ cup	granulated sugar
3 Tbsp	lemon juice
Pinch	each cinnamon and nutmeg

- In a large mixing bowl, cream the butter and sugar. Add the flour, baking powder, and salt. Add the eggs, and beat well.

- Spread the batter in a greased 9″ springform pan. Place the peaches, skin-side up, in a pattern on top.

- Sprinkle with the granulated sugar. Add the lemon juice, cinnamon, and nutmeg.

- Bake at 350°F for 1 hour, or until the peaches are tender and the cake is golden.

Old-Fashioned Butterscotch Pie

{ MAKES 8 SERVINGS }

No one can resist the rich buttery goodness of this favorite dessert!

NUTRIENTS PER SERVING:
Calories: 288
Protein: 6 grams
Fat: 12 grams
Carbohydrate: 39 grams

¾ cup	brown sugar
2 Tbsp	all-purpose flour
1¾ cups	milk (half evaporated)
1 Tbsp	butter (approx.)
2	egg yolks, well beaten
1 tsp	vanilla
1	prebaked 9″ pie shell

• In a bowl, mix the sugar and flour. Stir in the milk.

• In a saucepan, cook over medium heat until thick.

• Remove from heat. Add the butter and egg yolks. Return to the heat, and cook for 2 minutes longer. Remove from heat.

• Stir in the vanilla; pour the mixture into the pie shell, and spread evenly. Top with meringue (recipe follows).

MERINGUE

2	egg whites
¼ cup	granulated sugar

• In a bowl, beat the egg whites until soft peaks form. Very gradually beat in the sugar until the mixture is stiff. Spread evenly over the filling. Bake at 425°F for 4 to 5 minutes, or until the tips of the meringue are golden. Remove from the oven, and let cool. Chill before serving.

Ginger Pound Cake

{ MAKE 8 TO 12 SERVINGS }

Ginger adds a unique taste to this simple and delicious cake.

THIS RECIPE IS *FREE* OF THE FOLLOWING TRIGGERS

Caffeine ✓

Chocolate ✓

Citrus fruits ✓

Red wine ✓

Aged cheese ✓

MSG & nitrates ✓

Aspartame ✓

Nuts ✓

Onions & garlic ✓

Yeast ✓

NUTRIENTS PER SERVING
(when serving 12):

Calories: 426

Protein: 5 grams

Fat: 18 grams

Carbohydrate: 61 grams

1 cup	butter
1½ cups	fruit sugar
4	eggs
1 tsp	vanilla
2 cups	all-purpose flour
½ tsp	baking powder
¼ tsp	salt
1 cup	ginger marmalade

- In a large bowl, cream the butter with the sugar until light and fluffy. Add the eggs one at a time, beating well each time. Beat in the vanilla.

- In another bowl, combine the flour, baking powder, and salt. Blend the flour mixture into the butter mixture. Stir in the marmalade.

- Turn the batter into a greased and floured 9″ x 5″ or 8″ x 4″ loaf pan. Bake at 325°F for about 1¼ to 1½ hours, or until a tester inserted in the center comes out clean. Let cool in the pan, then turn out onto a rack to cool completely.

Maple Syrup Cake

{ MAKE 8 TO 12 SERVINGS }

Toasted coconut adds a delightful crunchiness to this moist maple cake.

NUTRIENTS PER SERVING
(when serving 12):

Calories: 220

Protein: 3 grams

Fat: 4 grams

Carbohydrate: 43 grams

SAUCE

1 cup	maple syrup
¾ cup	water
2 tsp	butter

CAKE

1 cup	all-purpose flour
½ cup	granulated sugar
1½ tsp	baking powder
½ tsp	salt
1	egg, well beaten
⅓ cup	milk
1 Tbsp	shortening
½ cup	shredded coconut

- In a saucepan, bring the syrup and water to a boil. Remove from the heat, and add the butter. Set aside.

- In a large bowl, mix together the flour, sugar, baking powder, and salt. Add the egg, milk, and shortening to make batter. Pour into a greased 8″ square pan.

- Pour the maple syrup sauce slowly over the batter. Sprinkle the coconut on top. Bake at 350°F for 35 minutes, or until a tester inserted in the center comes out clean. Let cool. Serve with whipped cream.

Cranberry Carrot Cake
WITH Cream Cheese Frosting

{ MAKES 12 TO 16 SERVINGS }

The cranberries in this recipe add a subtle tartness to this perennial favorite.

NUTRIENTS PER SERVING
(when serving 16):

Calories: 551

Protein: 6 grams

Fat: 27 grams

Carbohydrate: 71 grams

MAKE AHEAD: The cake can be baked a day in advance, wrapped in plastic wrap or foil, and stored at room temperature until ready to be frosted.

1½ cups	granulated sugar
1 cup	vegetable or canola oil
5	eggs, at room temperature
2½ cups	all-purpose flour
2¼ tsp	baking powder
2¼ tsp	cinnamon
2 tsp	baking soda
1 tsp	salt
3 cups	peeled and grated carrots
1½ cups	fresh cranberries

• In a large bowl, combine the sugar, oil, and eggs.

• Add the flour, baking powder, cinnamon, baking soda, and salt, and mix. Fold in the carrots and cranberries. Divide evenly between two 9″ round greased and floured cake pans.

• Bake at 300°F for about 45 minutes, or until a tester inserted in the center comes out clean. Let the cakes cool for 5 to 10 minutes in the pans before turning them out onto racks to cool completely. When cool, frost with Cream Cheese Frosting (recipe follows).

CREAM CHEESE FROSTING

½ cup	unsalted butter, at room temperature (1 stick)
8 oz	cream cheese
1 tsp	vanilla
4 cups	confectioners' sugar
¼ tsp	lemon zest

• Cream together the butter, cream cheese, and vanilla until fluffy.

• Beat in the sugar to make a smooth and spreadable consistency. Stir in the lemon zest. Frost the cooled Cranberry Carrot Cake.

Crème Brûlée with Rosemary

{ MAKES 4 SERVINGS }

This traditional French recipe is brought up to date with the addition of fragrant rosemary.

NUTRIENTS PER SERVING:

Calories: 580

Protein: 8 grams

Fat: 52 grams

Carbohydrate: 20 grams

6	egg yolks, at room temperature
⅓ cup	granulated sugar + additional for carmelizing
2 cups	35% cream
1/2 cup	homogenized milk
1 Tbsp	chopped fresh rosemary

♦ In a large stainless steel bowl, mix the egg yolks and sugar until well blended.

♦ In a heavy saucepan over medium-high heat, bring the cream, milk, and rosemary to a gentle boil, stirring occasionally. Remove from heat.

♦ Gradually, in a steady stream, pour the heated cream mixture into the egg yolks while constantly beating with a whisk. Let sit for 30 minutes at room temperature.

♦ Strain the mixture through a sieve into custard cups. Place the cups in a roasting pan. Fill the pan with boiling water so that it comes halfway up the sides of the cups.

♦ Place the roasting pan in the oven; bake at 350°F for 30 minutes. The custard is cooked when a thin knife inserted in the center comes out clean. Remove the cups from the roasting pan, and place in the refrigerator to cool (uncovered).

♦ Prior to serving, cover the custard in each cup with a generous layer of granulated sugar. Caramelize by placing the cups on a baking sheet under a preheated broiler. Watch carefully; remove once sugar has caramelized into a rich amber color.

Moltoff WITH Fresh Berry Compote

This fantastically light and elegant dessert will leave your guests clamoring for more!

THIS RECIPE IS *FREE* OF THE FOLLOWING TRIGGERS

Caffeine ✓

Chocolate ✓

Citrus fruits ✓

Red wine ✓

Aged cheese ✓

MSG & nitrates ✓

Aspartame ✓

Nuts ✓

Onions & garlic ✓

Yeast ✓

NUTRIENTS PER SERVING
(when serving 10):

Calories: 399

Protein: 5 grams

Fat: 3 grams

Carbohydrate: 88 grams

MAKE AHEAD: The moltoff, caramel, and berry compote can all be made a day in advance. Refrigerate overnight, and bring to room temperature before serving.

CARAMEL MOLTOFF

3 cups	granulated sugar
1 cup	water
10	egg whites
1 tsp	baking powder
2 Tbsp	unsalted butter
1–1½ cups	vanilla custard

♦ In a small saucepan over moderate heat, melt 2 cups of the sugar, stirring until darkened in color. Add the water, and let it reduce to syrup. Do not allow it to reduce too much. The caramel should not be too dark, and should thicken slightly as it cools.

♦ In a bowl, beat the egg whites with the remaining sugar and baking powder until soft peaks form. Add 1 tablespoon of the caramel and continue beating to incorporate. Set aside the remaining caramel.

♦ Butter the inside of a chilled round angel cake tube pan, and fill it with the egg white mixture. Place the pan in a deep baking or roasting pan filled with boiling water. Make sure the water comes halfway up the side of the tube pan.

♦ Bake at 375°F for 10 to 14 minutes, or until golden brown. Remove from the oven and the water bath, and let cool to room temperature. Invert onto a rack, and remove from the pan.

Fresh Berry Compote

1 cup	**water**
2 cups	**granulated sugar**
2 Tbsp	**orange liqueur (optional)**
2 cups	**each fresh blueberries, raspberries, and strawberries**
	Confectioners' sugar

- In a saucepan over medium-high heat, bring the water, sugar, and orange liqueur (if using) to a boil. Simmer until the mixture becomes syrup. Add the berries, and remove from heat. Let cool to room temperature.

- Reheat the remaining caramel. Slice the moltoff into sections, and place on individual dessert plates with a base of vanilla custard. Top with berry compote, and drizzle with the reheated caramel. Dust the edge of each plate with confectioners' sugar sifted through a sieve or fine strainer.

Lemon Curd WITH Shortbread Cookies AND Raspberry Coulis

{ MAKES 6 TO 8 SERVINGS }

The sweetness of the shortbread and raspberries is matched with the zesty taste of lemon in this delectable recipe.

THIS RECIPE IS *FREE* OF THE FOLLOWING TRIGGERS

Caffeine ✓

Chocolate ✓

Citrus fruits

Red wine ✓

Aged cheese ✓

MSG & nitrates ✓

Aspartame ✓

Nuts ✓

Onions & garlic ✓

Yeast ✓

NUTRIENTS PER SERVING
(when serving 8):

Calories: 494

Protein: 5 grams

Fat: 26 grams

Carbohydrate: 60 grams

MAKE AHEAD: The lemon curd can be prepared a day in advance; the raspberry coulis can be prepared several days in advance; and the shortbread cookies can be baked a day or two in advance. Store them individually in airtight containers in the refrigerator.

LEMON CURD

4	egg yolks, at room temperature
½ cup	granulated sugar
⅓ cup	fresh lemon juice
¼ cup	unsalted butter, at room temperature
Pinch	salt
2 tsp	lemon zest

◆ In a saucepan, whisk the egg yolks and sugar together.

◆ Add the lemon juice, butter, and salt.

◆ Cook over medium-low heat, stirring constantly, until thickened. Do not boil.

◆ Place the zest in a heat-resistant bowl. Place a strainer on top, and pour the egg mixture through the strainer. Discard what remains in the strainer.

◆ Allow the curd to cool. Store in a covered jar in the refrigerator if not using right away.

RASPBERRY COULIS

½ cup	water
1 Tbsp	cornstarch
1	pkg (about 15 oz) frozen, sweetened raspberries

◆ In a bowl, mix the water and cornstarch together.

◆ In a saucepan, simmer the raspberries over medium heat until all the frost is gone; quickly bring to a boil. Pour in the cornstarch and water mixture, stirring constantly.

◆ Cook for 1 minute, stirring constantly. Don't overcook or it will turn brown.

◆ Remove from heat, and let cool.

Shortbread Cookies

1½ cups	unsalted butter, at room temperature
½ cup	granulated sugar
4 cups	all-purpose flour, sifted 3 times

- In a mixing bowl, combine the butter and sugar, and beat until very light and fluffy.

- Place on a flat surface, and knead in the flour, a little at a time. On a lightly floured surface, form the dough into a flattened disc, and then roll it out to ¼″ thickness.

- Cut into shapes about 4″ in diameter. Gather the scraps, reroll, and cut into as many cookies as possible.

- Place the cookies on a cookie sheet lined with parchment paper. Bake at 350°F for approximately 10 to 12 minutes, or until lightly golden. Transfer to a rack to cool.

- Place each cookie on a plate. Drape 1 tablespoon lemon curd over a portion of cookie. Add a portion of the raspberry coulis over the curd. Garnish with a scattering of fresh raspberries or blueberries, if desired.

Mocha Mousse WITH Cinnamon Whipped Cream

{ MAKES 8 SERVINGS }

This rich dessert is quickly assembled. It contains decaffeinated espresso, but keep in mind that even "decaffeinated" coffees contain small amounts of caffeine.

NUTRIENTS PER SERVING:
Calories: 420
Protein: 5 grams
Fat: 32 grams
Carbohydrate: 28 grams

MAKE AHEAD: The mousse can be made earlier in the day and chilled for several hours.

5	eggs, at room temperature, separated
1 cup	granulated sugar
½ cup	unsalted butter, melted (1 stick)
¾ cup	decaffeinated espresso or instant
2 cups	35% cream, whipped until stiff

♦ In a bowl placed over a pan of simmering water or on top of a double boiler over simmering water, beat the egg yolks and sugar. Add the butter and whisk to combine. Continue to cook, whisking constantly, for 6 to 8 minutes, or until the mixture is thick like custard. Don't overcook the eggs or allow the water to boil, or the eggs will curdle.

♦ Remove from heat, and stir in the espresso. Cool to room temperature.

♦ In a large bowl, beat the egg whites until thick and fluffy and stiff peaks form. Gently fold them into the whipped cream.

♦ Stir about ⅓ of the egg-cream mixture thoroughly into the cooled coffee mixture. Fold the remaining egg-cream mixture into the coffee mixture until thoroughly blended.

♦ Pour into 8 dessert dishes or martini glasses. Chill for several hours. Serve with a dollop of Cinnamon Whipped Cream (recipe follows).

CINNAMON WHIPPED CREAM

3 Tbsp	granulated sugar
1 tsp	cinnamon
1 cup	35% cream

♦ In a small bowl, mix the sugar and cinnamon together.

♦ In a large chilled bowl, whip the cream until frothy. Add the sugar mixture, and whip until medium stiff peaks form. Serve dollops on top of Mocha Mousse.

Whole Wheat Doughnuts

{ MAKES ABOUT 4 DOZEN DOUGHNUTS }

The whole wheat flour in these doughnuts adds a nice texture. They're great for dunking in coffee or tea.

THIS RECIPE IS *FREE* OF THE FOLLOWING TRIGGERS

Caffeine ✓

Chocolate ✓

Citrus fruits ✓

Red wine ✓

Aged cheese ✓

MSG & nitrates ✓

Aspartame ✓

Nuts ✓

Onions & garlic ✓

Yeast ✓

NUTRIENTS PER SERVING:
Calories: 211
Protein: 2 grams
Fat: 15 grams
Carbohydrate: 17 grams

2½ cups	all-purpose flour
2½ cups	whole wheat flour
2 tsp	each baking soda, baking powder, and cream of tartar
3	eggs
1½ cups	granulated sugar
1 tsp	vanilla
1 tsp	nutmeg
1 tsp	salt
½ tsp	ginger
¼ cup	butter
1½ cups	milk
	Sugar and cinnamon (optional)

♦ In a large bowl, mix together the flours, baking soda, baking powder, and cream of tartar. Set aside.

♦ In another large bowl, beat together the eggs, sugar, vanilla, nutmeg, salt, and ginger until thick.

♦ Melt the butter, and add it to the milk. Add milk mixture and the flour mixture alternately to the egg mixture, beating after each addition just until blended.

♦ Cover the dough, and refrigerate for 2 to 3 hours or overnight.

♦ Roll it out on a floured board to ½″ thickness. Cut with a floured doughnut cutter. Deep fry at 375°F until golden brown on both sides. Drain on a paper towel. Roll in a sugar and cinnamon mixture, if desired.

Carob Chip Cookies

{ MAKES ABOUT 60 COOKIES }

If chocolate is a trigger, try these delectable carob chip cookies. Kids—and adults—love them.

NUTRIENTS PER SERVING:
Calories: 63
Protein: 1 gram
Fat: 3 grams
Carbohydrate: 8 grams

1⅔ cups	all-purpose flour
2 tsp	baking powder
½ tsp	baking soda
½ tsp	salt
⅔ cup	brown sugar
½ cup	margarine
1	egg
⅓ cup	corn syrup
1 tsp	vanilla (optional)
1 cup	carob chips

♦ In a mixing bowl, sift together the flour, baking powder, baking soda, and salt.

♦ In another bowl, cream together the sugar, margarine, egg, corn syrup, and vanilla (if using). Add the dry ingredients to the creamed mixture. Add the carob chips, and mix gently with your fingers.

♦ Drop teaspoonfuls well apart on a greased cookie sheet. Bake at 350°F for 10 to 12 minutes, or until golden brown. Cool on the cookie sheet for a few minutes, then remove to racks to cool completely.

No-Bake Carob-Oatmeal Macaroons

{ MAKES ABOUT 2 TO 3 DOZEN }

THIS RECIPE IS *FREE* OF THE FOLLOWING TRIGGERS

Caffeine ✓

Chocolate ✓

Citrus fruits ✓

Red wine ✓

Aged cheese ✓

MSG & nitrates ✓

Aspartame ✓

Nuts ✓

Onions & garlic ✓

Yeast ✓

NUTRIENTS PER SERVING
(1 macaroon when recipe makes 3 dozen).

Calories: 112

Protein: 1 gram

Fat: 4 grams

Carbohydrate: 18 grams

These yummy treats can be ready in less than 15 minutes.

2 cups	**granulated sugar**
½ cup	**shortening**
½ cup	**carob powder**
½ cup	**milk (or milk substitute)**
3 cups	**rolled oats**
½ cup	**shredded coconut or raisins**

◆ In a large saucepan, mix the sugar, shortening, carob powder, and milk. Boil the mixture until it bubbles.

◆ Remove from heat, and add the oats and coconut or raisins. Mix well, and drop by tablespoonfuls onto cookie sheets covered with waxed paper.

Almond Crescents

{ MAKES ABOUT 6 DOZEN COOKIES }

These crescent-shaped treats have the mellow flavor of almonds and confectioners' sugar. They're perfect with herbal tea.

THIS RECIPE IS *FREE* OF THE FOLLOWING TRIGGERS

Caffeine ✓

Chocolate ✓

Citrus fruits ✓

Red wine ✓

Aged cheese ✓

MSG & nitrates ✓

Aspartame ✓

Nuts

Onions & garlic ✓

Yeast ✓

NUTRIENTS PER SERVING:
Calories: 64
Protein: 1 gram
Fat: 4 grams
Carbohydrate: 6 grams

2¼ cups	flour
½ tsp	salt
1¼ cups	softened butter
1 cup	confectioners' sugar + additional for sprinkling
2 tsp	vanilla
1 cup	ground almonds

◆ In a bowl, stir together the flour and salt. In a separate bowl, cream the butter; beat in the sugar and vanilla. Gradually add the dry ingredients to the creamed mixture. Add the almonds.

◆ Form into 1″ balls; shape into crescents. Bake on an ungreased cookie sheet at 325°F for 12 to 15 minutes, or until lightly browned. Sprinkle with confectioners' sugar while still warm.

Icebox Ginger Snaps

{ MAKES ABOUT 5 DOZEN COOKIES }

Memories of childhood will abound when the warm and wonderful aroma of baking ginger snaps fills your kitchen.

THIS RECIPE IS *FREE* OF THE FOLLOWING TRIGGERS

Caffeine ✓

Chocolate ✓

Citrus fruits ✓

Red wine ✓

Aged cheese ✓

MSG & nitrates ✓

Aspartame ✓

Nuts ✓

Onions & garlic ✓

Yeast ✓

NUTRIENTS PER SERVING:
Calories: 72
Protein: 1 gram
Fat: 4 grams
Carbohydrate: 8 grams

1 cup	shortening
⅔ cup	molasses
⅓ cup	brown sugar
3 cups	all-purpose flour
2 tsp	ginger
1 tsp	cinnamon
½ tsp	salt
½ tsp	baking soda
½ tsp	cloves

♦ In a bowl, cream together the shortening, molasses, and brown sugar. In a separate bowl, mix the flour, ginger, cinnamon, salt, baking soda, and cloves. Add to the creamed mixture. Shape the dough into a roll 2 inches in diameter. Wrap in waxed paper and refrigerate until firm, about 4 hours.

♦ Cut the dough into ¼″ slices. Bake on a greased baking sheet at 400°F for 5 to 7 minutes, or until lightly browned. Let cool for a few minutes on the baking sheet; transfer to racks to cool completely.

Beverages

Mint Julep

On a warm summer's evening, this traditional southern beverage's tangy/sweet flavor is the perfect refresher. Substitute apple juice for the lemon juice if citrus is a trigger.

THIS RECIPE IS *FREE* OF THE FOLLOWING TRIGGERS

Caffeine ✓

Chocolate ✓

Citrus fruits

Red wine ✓

Aged cheese ✓

MSG & nitrates ✓

Aspartame ✓

Nuts ✓

Onions & garlic ✓

Yeast ✓

NUTRIENTS PER SERVING:
Calories: 176
Carbohydrate: 44 grams

1	bunch fresh mint
1½ cups	sugar
1 cup	lemon juice
½ cup	water
3 pints	ginger ale

♦ Discard the stems and injured leaves of the mint. In a bowl, cover the good leaves with the sugar, lemon juice, and water. Let stand for 30 minutes. Pour over ice in a large pitcher. Add the ginger ale.

Peppermint Cooler

{ MAKES ABOUT 8 SERVINGS }

This frosty beverage is excellent served as a dessert. It's rich in calcium, too!

NUTRIENTS PER SERVING:
Calories: 261
Protein: 10 grams
Fat: 9 grams
Carbohydrate: 35 grams

8 cups	milk
½ cup	sugar
1 tsp	peppermint extract (or more to taste)
	Vanilla ice cream
	Peppermint stick candy, crushed
	Mint leaves

♦ In a large saucepan, heat the milk and sugar until the sugar is dissolved. Let cool, then chill.

♦ When chilled, add the peppermint extract. To serve, place a scoop of vanilla ice cream in a tall glass, and pour milk mixture over it. Garnish with crushed peppermint candy and a mint leaf.

Migraine Mellower

{ MAKES 1 SERVING }

A soothing beverage with the medicinal attributes of ginger.

THIS RECIPE IS *FREE* OF THE FOLLOWING TRIGGERS

Caffeine ✓

Chocolate ✓

Citrus fruits ✓

Red wine ✓

Aged cheese ✓

MSG & nitrates ✓

Aspartame ✓

Nuts ✓

Onions & garlic ✓

Yeast ✓

NUTRIENTS PER SERVING:
Calories: 80
Carbohydrate: 20 grams

⅓ cup	apple juice
½ cup	ginger ale or ginger beer
	candied ginger (optional)

◆ In a tall glass, combine the apple juice and ginger ale. Garnish with a thin slice of candied ginger, if desired.

Frosty Fruit Punch

Try making a frozen version of this punch. Your children will love the delicious slushy treat.

NUTRIENTS PER 1-CUP SERVING
Calories: 120
Carbohydrate: 30 grams

1	can frozen unsweetened apple juice concentrate
1½ cups	unsweetened grape juice
¼–½ cup	fresh squeezed lemon juice
¼ cup	cranberry juice concentrate (optional)

TO MAKE THE BASE:

• Combine the apple juice concentrate, grape and lemon juice, and cranberry juice concentrate, if using.

TO MAKE THE PUNCH:

• Add 1 can of club soda to 1 cup of the base.

{ **KITCHEN POINTER:** To make a frozen drink for a child's lunch, substitute water for the club soda. A 6-oz plastic container of this mixture can be frozen and added to your child's lunch box. It will keep the lunch cool and be ready to drink by lunchtime. }

Hot Spiced Punch

In winter, welcome your guests with this special warming drink.

NUTRIENTS PER 1-CUP SERVING
Calories: 172
Carbohydrate: 43 grams

2	cinnamon sticks
6	whole cloves
½ cup	brown sugar
2 cups	cranberry juice
8 cups	apple juice

◆ Place the spices and sugar in a percolator basket, and pour the juices into the pot. Percolate for 5 minutes. May also be simmered on the stove top.

Mulled Cider

This old-fashioned favorite is perfect for a festive holiday gathering or a wintry night with the family.

THIS RECIPE IS *FREE* OF THE FOLLOWING TRIGGERS

Caffeine ✓

Chocolate ✓

Citrus fruits ✓

Red wine ✓

Aged cheese ✓

MSG & nitrates ✓

Aspartame ✓

Nuts ✓

Onions & garlic ✓

Yeast ✓

NUTRIENTS PER SERVING:
Calories: 280
Carbohydrate: 70 grams

1	large apple
20	cloves
4 cups	apple juice or apple cider
½	whole nutmeg
5	short cinnamon sticks
1 tsp	ground ginger
¾ cup	brown sugar

◆ Stud the apple with the cloves. Place in a pot. Pour in the apple juice. Break the nutmeg and one cinnamon stick, and add them to the pot along with the ginger. Simmer for 30 minutes. Add the sugar. Strain into mugs. Garnish each mug with a cinnamon stick and an apple slice.

Bibliography

Bickerstaff, E.R. *Neurological complications of oral contraceptives*. Oxford: Clarendon Press, 1975.

Bousser, M.G., and H. Massiou. "Migraine in the reproductive cycle." In J. Olesen. et al, *The Headaches*. New York: Raven Press, 1993.

Critchley, Macdonald. "Migraine: From Cappadocia to Queen Square." in *Background to Migraine* (ed.) Robert Smith. New York: Springer-Verlag, 1967.

Edmeads, John. "History of migraine treatment." *Can. J Clin Pharmacol 1999*; 6 (suppl A), Autumn: 5A–8A.

Edmeads J., H. Findlay, P. Tugwell et al. "Impact of migraine and tension-type headache on lifestyle, consulting behaviour, and medication use: a Canadian population survey." *Can. J Neurol Sci 1993*; 20:131–137.

Epstein, M.T., J.M. Hockaday, and T.D. Hockaday. "Migraine and reproductive hormones throughout the menstrual cycle." *The Lancet 1975*; 1(7906):543–548.

Ferrari, M.D. The Economic Burden of Migraine to Society. *Pharmacoeconomics 1998*; 13:667–676.

Gilmour, H., and K. Wilkins. *Statistics Canada, Health Reports 2001*; Vol. 12, No. 2. Catalogue 82-003.

Goadsby, Peter, et al. *Headache in Clinical Practice*, Oxford: Isis Medical Media Ltd., 1998.

Hu, X.H., et al. "Burden of Migraine in the United States: Disability and Economic Costs." *Archives of International Medicine 1999*; 159: 813-818.

Kudrow, L. "The relationship of headache frequency to hormone use in migraine." *Headache 1975*; 15 (Apr):36–40.

Lipton, R.B., and W.F. Stewart. "Migraine in the United States: Epidemiology and Health Care Use." *Neurology 1993*; 43 (suppl 3):6–10.

McKim, A. Elizabeth. "Ancient Migraine." *Headlines 8-3*, 1999: 1–5.

O'Brien, B., R. Goeree, and D. Streiner. "Prevalence of Migraine Headache in Canada: A Population-Based Survey." *Int J Epidemiol 1994*; 23:1020–1026.

Osterhaus J.T., R.J. Townsend, B. Gandek et al. "Measuring the functional status and well-being of patients with migraine headache." *Headache 1994*; 34:337–343.

Pryse-Phillips W., H. Findlay, P. Tugwell et al. "A Canadian Population Survey on the Clinical, Epidemiologic and Societal Impact of Migraine and Tension-Type Headache." *Can J Neurol Sci 1992*; 19:333–339.

Silberstein, S.D. "Migraine and women: the link between headache and hormones." *Postgraduate Medicine 1995*; 97(4):147–153.

Silberstein, S.D., and R.B. Lipton. "Headache epidemiology: emphasis on migraine." *Neurology Clinics 1996*; 14:421–434.

Simon, Maurice (ed.) *The Babylonian Talmud: Seder Nashim Vol. 3*. London: Soncino, 1936.

South, Valerie. *Migraine*. Toronto: Key Porter Books, 1994.

Stewart, W.F., R.B. Lipton et al. "Prevalence of migraine headache in the United States: Relation to age, income, race and other socio-demographic factors." *JAMA 1992*; 267(1):64–69.

List of Resources

WORLD HEADACHE ALLIANCE

More than 40 headache organizations from more than 30 nations worldwide have recently come together to form the unprecedented global cooperative World Headache Alliance.

The alliance aims to improve the lives of people with headache throughout the world by sharing information among existing headache organizations and by fostering the development of new headache organizations in areas where none currently exists. Together, these organizations seek to increase the awareness and understanding of headache as a public health concern with profound social and economic impact.

World Headache Alliance (WHA) member organizations are working side by side today with the best headache researchers, scientists, and clinicians. WHA is working closely with the professionally based International Headache Society (www.i-h-s.org) toward jointly fostering relationships with the World Health Organization in Geneva, Switzerland, to ensure that headache disorders receive full attention worldwide.

For up-to-the-minute information, check out the World Headache Alliance's web site at www.ihaveaheadache.com. For more information on WHA, you can also contact:

World Headache Alliance
208 Lexington Road
Oakville, ON
Canada L6H 6L6
(905) 257-6229 Fax: (905) 257-6239

Lay (Patient-Based) Migraine Organizations
United States

The American Council for Headache Education (ACHE)

19 Mantua Road

Mount Royal, NJ 08061

(856) 423-0258 Fax: (856) 423-0082

Toll-Free: 1-800-255-ACHE

E-mail: achehq@talley.com www.achenet.org

The American Council for Headache Education is a nonprofit partnership of patients and health professionals dedicated to advancing the treatment and management of headache and to raising public awareness of headache as a valid, biologically based illness. ACHE's goal is to help sufferers gain more control over all aspects of their lives—medical, social, and economic. ACHE members receive the quarterly newsletter *Headache* as well as free access to an expanding series of brochures, videos, and books covering a wide variety of topics relating to headache. ACHE has established a growing national network of headache support groups and it has gone online, giving members expanded access to headache information and support via Prodigy, America OnLine, and the Internet.

ACHE is affiliated with the American Headache Society (AHS), an organization of more than a 1,000 physicians allied with health professionals and research scientists. If you are not already receiving proper medical care for your headache, ACHE can supply you with a complete list of affiliated AHS physician members in your area. An Access to Care Committee has also been founded to explore problems encountered by sufferers attempting to obtain specialized services and medications.

MAGNUM, The National Migraine Association

113 South Saint Asaph Street

Suite 100

Alexandria, Va 22414-3119

(703) 739-9384 Fax: (703) 739-2342

E-mail: magnumnonprofit@hotmail.com

www.migraines.org

Migraine Association of the Upper Midwest, Inc.

1911 Ryan West

Roseville, Mn 55113

(651) 636-2564 Fax: (651) 636-0663

E-mail: pkirbyrsvle@uswest.net

National Headache Foundation

5252 North Western Avenue

Chicago, IL 60625

(312) 878-7715 Toll-free: 1-800-843-2256

www.headaches.org

Canada

The Migraine Association of Canada

365 Bloor St. East, Suite 1912

Toronto, ON M2W 3L4

(416) 920-4916 Fax: (416) 920-3677

Toll-free membership information: 1-800-663-3557

24-hour recorded information: (416) 920-4917

E-mail: support@migraine.ca www.migraine.ca

An important step in managing migraine involves keeping abreast of current developments in migraine treatment and research. It is also important for migraine sufferers to band together in sharing information and in promoting awareness of the serious nature of migraine. Sufferers can look to The Migraine Association of Canada for this assistance. Founded in 1974 by Rosemary Dudley, The Migraine Association is the only national charity solely committed to providing quality services and programs to millions of people afflicted with migraine.

Through The Migraine Association's educational literature, millions learn about this medical disorder and about ways of gaining the upper hand in the struggle against migraine's debilitating symptoms. Members of the association receive a comprehensive information package upon enrollment, along with a yearly subscription to the association's newsletter. Information contained in the quarterly newsletter will appeal to both the newly diagnosed and the longtime sufferer. Details on the latest in migraine research, theories, and treatment options are included. Members share victories and failures in their treatment strategies, as well as tips on coping with migraine. Books and videos are sold through the association as well.

The Migraine Association of Canada's awareness events ensure that migraine is recognized as a serious medical disorder. Improved understanding of migraine spawns new interest in medical research; the mobilization of funds for the development of new treatments; and an enhanced concern for migraine sufferers from doctors, other health care professionals, government, the media, and the general public.

Fondation Québécoise de la Migraine et des Céphalées
(Quebec Migraine and Headache Foundation)
1575 Boulevard Henri Bourassa W., Suite 240
Montreal, PQ H3M 3A9
(514) 331-8207 Fax: (514) 331-8809
E-mail: tete@fqmc.qc.ca www.fqmc.qc.ca
(Service mainly in French, but English language
brochures are available)

Help for Headaches
647 Ouellette Avenue, Suite #104
Windsor, ON N9A 4J4
(519) 252-3727 Fax: (519) 252-5537
E-mail: brent@headache-help.org www.headache-help.org

WEB SITES

American Academy of Neurology (AAN): www.aan.com
Canadian Medical Association Journal: www.cma.ca/cmaj
Neurology (journal of AAN): www.neurology.org
Ronda's Migraine Page: www.migrainepage.com/
Jama Migraine: www.ama-assn.org/special/migraine/migraine
Women's Health Interactive:
www.womens-health.com/health_centre/headache/migraine.html

Index

h

halibut:
  Baked Halibut with Dill Crust and Red Pepper Sauce, 94
headache. *see also* migraine
  cluster, 6
  medication-induced, 6
  tension, 3
Help for Headaches, 172
honey:
  Honey-Roasted Lamb Tenderloin with Green Asparagus and Plantain Mash, 80–81
  Lemon Sole with Oranges and Honey, 95
  Roast Duck with Spiced Honey, 76
hummus, 32
hypnotherapy, 16

l

lamb:
  Honey-Roasted Lamb Tenderloin with Green Asparagus and Plantain Mash, 80–81
  Quick Lamb Patties, 82
leek:
  Curried Winter Vegetable Soup, 43
  Vichyssoise, 42
lemon:
  Lemon Curd with Shortbread Cookies and Raspberry Coulis, 150–151
lentils:
  Curried Winter Vegetable Soup, 43

m

MAGNUM (The National Migraine Association), 170
mango:
  Grilled Salmon Steaks with Mango Strawberry Cilantro Chutney, 92
  Pan-Seared River Trout with Cucumber and Baby Shrimp Salsa, 93
marinades. *see also* sauces
  Balsamic Vinegar and Garlic Marinade, 97
  Orange-Sesame Marinade, 97
  sesame oil and soy sauce, 58–59
massage, 16
meals, skipped, 22
meat and poultry:
  Chicken Kabobs with Homemade Barbecue Sauce, 72
  Curried Chicken with Peaches and Coconut, 69
  Homestyle Chicken and Rice Casserole, 67
  Honey-Roasted Lamb Tenderloin with Green Asparagus and Plantain Mash, 80–81
  Japanese Glazed Chicken, 70
  Phyllo-Wrapped Chicken with Mushrooms and Spinach in Citron Vodka Sauce, 74–75
  Poached Chicken with Wild Rice and Baby Vegetables, 73
  Pork Tenderloin with Fresh Tomato Sauce, 79
  Quick Lamb Patties, 82
  Roast Duck with Spiced Honey, 76
  Simple Chicken Kiev, 68
  Swedish Meatballs, 77
  Sweet-and-Sour Pork Chops, 78
meatless main courses. *see vegetarian entrees*
medication, for migraine, 8–9, 14–15
medication-induced (rebound) headache, 6
menopause, migraine and, 7
migraine:
  amines and, 18–19
  avoiding, 23
  causes of, 4
  children and, 7–9
  complementary therapies, 15–16
  diagnosis of, 10–13
  managing, 14–16
  medication for, 8–9, 14–15
  resources, list of, 169–172
  symptoms of, 3, 10–11
  triggers, 8, 11–13, 17–21
  types of, 4–5
  women and, 6–7, 12
The Migraine Association of Canada, 171
Migraine Association of the Upper Midwest, Inc., 170
mint:
  Middle Eastern Salad, 47
  Mint Anglaise, Roasted Pears with, 136–137
  Mint Julep, 161
MSG (monosodium glutamate), as trigger, 18, 20
mushrooms. *see also* portobello mushroom; shiitake mushroom
  Cream of Mushroom Soup, 39
  Homestyle Chicken and Rice Casserole, 67
  Mushrooms and Rice, 108
  Phyllo-Wrapped Chicken with Mushrooms and Spinach in Citron Vodka Sauce, 74–75
  Roasted Wild Mushroom Veggie Burgers, 57
  Shiitake Pierogies with Sweet Ginger Sauce, 33
mustard:
  Dijon, and raspberry vinegar dressing, 48–49
  Grilled Gravlax with Mustard Dill Sauce, 36
  Yellowfin Tuna with Maple Mustard Sauce and Coriander Oil, 86–87

n

National Headache Foundation (MAGNUM), 171
The National Migraine Association, 170